I0842280


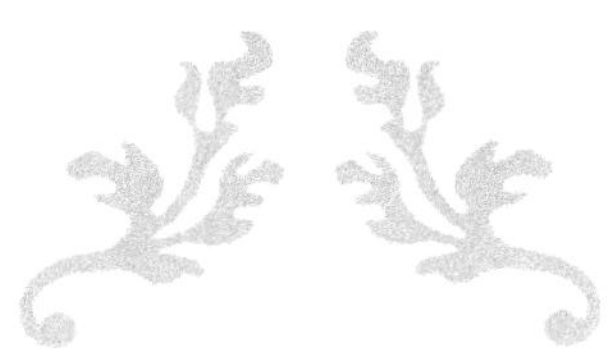

# THE GALVESTON DIET:

## Delicious and Healthy Recipes for Losing Weight and Living Well

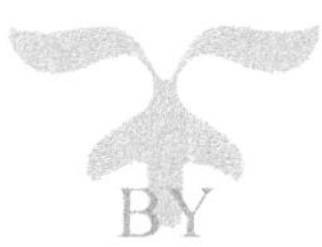

BY

## DR DEBORAH MARIN

Copyright © **by Dr Deborah Marin 2023. All rights reserved.**

Before the document is duplicated or reproduced in any manner, the publisher consents must be gained. Therefore, the contents within can neither be stored electrically, transferred, nor kept in a database.

Neither in part nor full can the document to copied, scanned, faxed, or retained without approval from the publisher or creator.

# TABLE OF CONTENTS


*INTRODUCTION*...................................................................4

*CHAPTER 1*

THE BASICS OF THE GALVESTON DIET ....................................6

GALVESTON DIET SAMPLE MENU .........................................11

GALVESTON DIET HELP PEOPLE TO LOSE WEIGHT..............12

THE 1,500-CALORIE DIET......................................................15

GM DIET ...............................................................................20

*CHAPTER 2*

UNDERSTANDING MACRONUTRIENTS....................................28

FUNCTIONS OF MACRONUTRIENTS .......................................31

COMPARING MACRONUTRIENTS AND MICRONUTRIENTS .33

FOOD SOURCES FOR FAT, PROTEIN, AND CARBOHYDRATES
...............................................................................................38

*CHAPTER 3*

EATING FOR MAXIMUM HEALTH ...........................................40

HOW TO FAMILIARIZE A HEALTHY DIET TO YOUR LIFE .......46

ADVICE FOR EATING WELL IN THE REAL WORLD .................48

*CHAPTER 4*

GROCERY SHOPPING AND MEAL PLANNING .....................51

*CHAPTER 5*

EXERCISE AND FITNESS........................................................57

ADVANTAGES OF EXERCISE ....................................61

WAYS THAT EXERCISING CAN MAKE YOU HAPPIER AND
HEALTHIER. ........................................................64

CREATE A SMART OBJECTIVE. ..............................68

THE BEST METHODS FOR STAYING IN SHAPE AFTER 40 ......73

HOW TO GET MOTIVATED TO EXERCISE ..............76

ADVICE FOR WEIGHT LOSS ..................................81

ADVICE FOR EATING WELL ..................................82

*CHAPTER 6*

LIVING A HEALTHY LIFESTYLE ............................83

ADVICE FOR REGULAR HEALTHY EATING ............84

PHYSICAL AND MENTAL HEALTH BENEFITS OF EXERCISE....86

MENTAL HEALTH....................................................88

STEER CLEAR OF RISKY SEXUAL CONDUCT.............92

STAY AWAY FROM OTHER RISKY ACTIVITIES.......93

FOODS FOR STABILIZING YOUR BLOOD VESSELS AND HEART
........................................................................95

*FINAL SUMMARY*..............................................107

# *INTRODUCTION*

"Welcome to The Galveston Diet, a science-based strategy for long-term health and wellness. A comprehensive program for healthy eating called the Galveston Diet emphasizes whole foods with little processing. By offering a balanced and wholesome meal plan and pointers and tricks to keep you on track, the diet is created to assist you in reaching your health goals. You'll be able to keep a healthy weight, lower your risk of developing chronic diseases, and gain the advantages of having excellent health by adhering to the Galveston Diet.

Are you sick of yo-yo dieting and the constant battle to keep a healthy weight? Do you wish to enhance your general health and well-being but are confused by the conflicting information available? The Galveston Diet is the only option.

A strategy for long-term weight loss and optimum health, the Galveston Diet is supported by science. This program is specifically tailored for women and addresses the particular hormonal and metabolic challenges they face, based on the most recent research in nutrition and metabolism. For those seeking to enhance their wellness and health, the Galveston Diet is the ideal option. The diet emphasizes whole foods with little processing and offers a well-balanced, nutrient-dense meal plan. It also provides advice on how to stay on track and accomplish your health objectives. You'll be able to maintain a healthy weight by following the Galveston Diet, lower your risk of developing chronic diseases, and benefit from having excellent health.

You can learn about the Galveston Diet's principles and how to apply them to your daily life in this book. You will learn about useful tools to change your body, such as nutrient-dense meal plans and self-care techniques, and you will be guided through the science behind the Galveston Diet, dispelling common misconceptions and sharing the most recent research on the intricate connection between nutrition and health.

The Galveston Diet offers suggestions on how to apply these ideas in real-world situations, including meal plans, shopping lists, and recipes. The balance of hormones and stress management are two other crucial areas of women's health that are covered in the book. The Galveston Diet offers a sustainable and individualized approach to achieving your goals, regardless of whether you want to lose weight, increase your energy, or just feel your best. Start your journey to optimal health today and join the thousands of women who have already changed their lives with this program based on scientific evidence.

The health and diet of women are the main topics of this book. The book suggests adopting a new way of life based on the ideas of the Mediterranean diet, intermittent fasting, and a high-fat, low-carb strategy.

"We hope that this book has given you the knowledge and resources you need to start following The Galveston Diet and embarking on your path to long-lasting health and wellness. We appreciate that you decided on The Galveston Diet and wish you the best of luck on your journey. Let's start now!"

# CHAPTER 1

## THE BASICS OF THE GALVESTON DIET

Inflammation-fighting diets are here to stay. The Galveston Diet, a new anti-inflammatory eating plan made especially for women, has gained a lot of popularity lately.

The Galveston Diet was created for women who want to prevent weight gain and may be having difficulty losing weight during these stages of life. This includes women who are in any stage of menopause, including per menopause. Additionally, it can help with typical hormonal side effects like brain fog, night sweats, and hot flashes. Their website claims to have 100,000 users in its community.

According to nutritionist Roxana Ehsani, RD, CSSD, LDN, "the diet is said to be an anti-inflammatory diet similar to the Mediterranean diet but also includes 16:8 intermittent fasting. For your information, that is when you eat for eight hours and then fast for the remaining sixteen hours of the day. The diet prohibits fried foods, vegetable oils, white flour, foods with high-fructose corn syrup, and processed foods with added sugar, artificial ingredients, colors, and flavorings.

According to Anya Rosen, RD, the founder of Birchwell, a virtual integrative health clinic, more and more middle-aged women are having difficulty losing weight and are beginning to understand that this is largely due to hormonal changes. This is why the diet is currently popular.

There are many similarities between the Galveston Diet and the ketogenic diet. The Galveston Diet is a high-fat, low-carb diet that consists of roughly 70% calories from fat, 20% calories from protein, and 9% calories from carbohydrates. The diet is currently in its low-carbohydrate phase. Depending on how much weight a person wants to lose, each person's duration will vary. The Galveston Diet differs from the keto diet in that you gradually increase your carbohydrate intake after a while in order to maintain ketosis, a metabolic state in which your body burns fat for energy instead of carbohydrates. The Galveston Diet differs from the ketogenic diet in that it prescribes the types of fat you should eat. It contains wholesome fats (such as olive oil, nuts, and seeds) while avoiding inflammatory ones (e.g., butter and red meat).

The Galveston Diet might be the healthier choice out of the two. "It supports better health than the traditional keto diet because it recognizes that the quality of the food matters just as much as the number of macronutrients."

What benefits and drawbacks does the Galveston Diet offer?

You don't have to count calories on the Galveston Diet, which may be more effective for some people. Furthermore, the diet avoids crash dieting and calorie restriction in favor of assisting you in forming long-term successful eating and exercise habits.

The 16:8 diet may discourage late-night eating or snacking if you're just starting it. On the other hand, it might lead some individuals to overeat during the feeding window in order to stave off hunger pangs at a later time when they shouldn't be eating.

Additionally, you can modify the Galveston Diet to make it suitable for vegans and vegetarians. The diet itself does not forbid foods derived from animals, but it can be made vegetarian- or vegan-friendly.

The only drawback is that there have been no clinical trials or studies on this diet, so it's difficult to say for sure whether it works to reduce inflammation, menopause symptoms, or promote weight loss (unlike the Mediterranean diet, which can lower inflammation). However, if the reviews are any indication, a lot of the women who tried this diet succeeded in losing weight and felt healthier and more confident than they had in the past.

To be honest, it is pretty safe to try the diet. Just be sure to consult your doctor before beginning, particularly if you have diabetes, immunosuppression, or a history of disordered eating, as intermittent fasting is not advised if any of these apply to you.

Evidence on the methods of the Galveston Diet suggests that its anti-inflammatory, intermittent fasting approach may aid menopausal people in losing weight more successfully than calorie restriction alone. One diet cannot work for everyone, and there is no specific research on this diet.

The three main areas the programs concentrate on to assist with hormone balancing and weight loss during menopause are:

• Intermittent fasting: In a 24-hour period, people may eat only within a time window of 8 hours and need to fast for the remaining 16 hours.
• Nutrition with anti-inflammatory properties: The diet promotes the consumption of foods with inherent antioxidant and anti-inflammatory properties. This might support the digestive system and improve how well the body functions.
• Refocus on fuel: The programs stress overcoming what they refer to as the "addiction to sugar and processed carbohydrates" and reorienting toward more nutrient-dense sources of carbohydrates.
I advise anyone starting a diet to familiarize themselves with these ideas and get ready to alter their perspective and eating behavior.

The Galveston Diet emphasizes avoiding processed foods and foods with added sugar while consuming naturally anti-inflammatory and antioxidant-rich foods. Suitable foods for the diet include:

**Proteins**
- Salmon
- Eggs
- quinoa
- Greek yogurt
- Lean grass-fed beef
- Lean chicken
- Lean turkey
- Nitrate-free deli meats.

**Fruits and vegetables**
- Spinach

- Tomatoes
- Cucumbers
- celery, broccoli
- cauliflower, blueberries
- raspberries,
- Strawberries.

**Fats**
- Avocado
- extra virgin olive oil
- walnuts
- pecans
- almonds
- sesame seeds
- sunflower seeds
- Pine nuts.

**What Not To Do**
The diet also advises staying away from the following items:
• refined flours and grains; processed or refined carbohydrate foods like pizza, chips, and white pasta;
• foods with artificial flavors, colors, preservatives, and high fructose corn syrup; processed meats with nitrates, such as sausages, burgers, and salami; fried foods; sugary drinks and sodas; sugar or artificial sweeteners added to hot drinks; oils that may be considered inflammatory, such as canola and vegetable;

# GALVESTON DIET SAMPLE MENU

You can check out the provided six-day meal plan if you're interested in learning more about this diet.

Day 1: Breakfast: Scrambled eggs with tomatoes, spinach, and mushrooms cooked in olive oil, along with a cup of berries; Lunch: Grilled chicken breast with mixed greens and avocado cooked in olive oil. Dinner will be shrimp over zoodles. Snacks will be cashews and strawberries.

Day 2: For breakfast, a Greek yogurt bowl with berries, almond butter, and chia seeds; for lunch, ground beef-stuffed Portobello mushrooms; and for dinner, spaghetti squash with a veggie marinara sauce.
• Snack: celery and hummus

Day 3: For breakfast, have a blueberry smoothie with collagen and spinach leaves; for lunch, have a beef burger without a bun over grilled eggplant, lettuce, tomatoes, avocado, and onion; for dinner, have roasted salmon with asparagus and cauliflower rice; and for snacks, have cheese slices and sugar snap peas.

Day 4: For breakfast, have plain Greek yogurt with chia seeds, chopped walnuts, and raspberries; for lunch, have a spinach salad with grilled chicken, feta, vinegar, and olive oil; for dinner, have baked salmon with roasted asparagus; and for supper, have two hard-boiled eggs with everything-but-the-bagels seasoning.

Day 5: Vegetable omelet cooked in avocado oil for breakfast, served with berries; bell peppers baked with lean ground turkey for lunch; zucchini topped with diced avocado for dinner.

Day 6 Breakfast: Chia seed pudding with crushed almonds and blueberries Lunch: Salad with spring mix, grilled shrimp, red onions, avocado, and olive oil drizzle Dinner: Cauliflower rice taco bowl with lean ground beef, peppers, and guacamole Snack: Celery sticks with almond butter Day 7 Breakfast: Chia seed pudding with crushed almonds and blueberries

## GALVESTON DIET HELP PEOPLE TO LOSE WEIGHT

As opposed to counting calories, which is the main focus of many weight loss diets, the Galveston Diet uses a different approach to weight loss.

Although there are no specific studies on the Galveston Diet itself, a lot of research has been done on some of the fundamental ideas behind the eating plan. These include the benefits of consuming foods that increase feelings of satiety or fullness as well as intermittent fasting.

For instance, it suggests that the body makes up for a calorie deficit after dieting, reaching a fixed point where people either stop losing weight or gain it back. The authors contend that it is more advantageous to comprehend how foods affect satiety and energy balance.

The review adopts the Galveston Diet's philosophy, which places an emphasis on how food can affect menopausal weight gain through inflammation and hormone changes.

Intermittent fasting is a key component of the Galveston Diet, which research indicates may be beneficial for weight loss.

No matter how many calories they consumed overall, participants in the 27 studies on intermittent fasting for weight loss lost 0.8% to 13% of their starting weight. Studies that lasted between two and twelve weeks also revealed a 4.3% decrease in body mass index and stable or lessened hunger symptoms.

Another 115 obese women showed that, over a 3-month period, carbohydrate restriction and intermittent fasting led to greater body fat loss than a diet with fewer calories.

One used the Galveston Diet's 16-hour fasting window as a weight-loss intervention for adults with abdominal obesity. After three months, their waist size shrunk by more than five centimeters.

Bearing in mind the readings above, there seems to be substantial suggestion that the Galveston Diet's method may be active for weight loss.

Other advantages

Due to its anti-inflammatory approach and intermittent fasting techniques, the Galveston Diet may have additional health advantages in addition to helping people lose weight.

Inflammation caused by adipose tissue in the body may be reduced by intermittent fasting (fat stores).

Intermittent fasting may help to stop insulin battle and diabetes, agreeing to the same reading.

## May lower the risk of some diseases.

The helpful anti-inflammatory properties of intermittent fasting may also help to stop prolonged circumstances such as metabolic syndrome and cardiovascular sickness. The damaging effects of oxidative stress, which produces the free radicals responsible for disease and aging, may also be mitigated by intermittent fasting. Intermittent fasting may help lower blood pressure, ward off diseases like cancer, and extend life.

## Could Raise Motivation

Some Galveston Diet program subscriptions include additional support and activity components, which might make people who are trying the diet feel more motivated to stick with it. Additionally, they might encourage people to exercise more frequently than usual. Both of these things may profit weight loss and over-all well-being.

## Drawbacks

The Galveston Diet's main potential drawback is that some people may find it difficult to adhere to and incorporate into their lifestyle.

## Cost

The subscription programs on the official diet website may be too expensive for people trying to lose weight on a tight budget. The price of some of the foods the program suggests, like grass-fed beef, may also be prohibitive. Additionally, depending on where they live, people might have trouble obtaining particular foods.

**Hunger during a fast**
Those who participate in the official programs may initially find fasting for 16 hours challenging.
If a person has their evening meal at 7 p.m. and has a time-restricted eating window of 8 hours, they are not allowed to eat again until 11 a.m. the next day. Some people might find it difficult to skip breakfast or eat it much later than usual if they do this.
The 16-hour fasting window can be flexible, so someone could eat their evening meal at 5 p.m. and breakfast at 9 a.m., which may be more convenient for some. Alternatively, if someone prefers, they can skip their evening meal and just eat their breakfast and lunch as usual.

**Socializing**
It might be more difficult for someone to socialize and eat out if they are restricted from consuming certain foods and beverages. For this reason, a person trying the diet may want to make advance plans and take social events into account.


# THE 1,500-CALORIE DIET
People who are attempting to lose weight may try the 1,500-calorie diet. People can create a calorie deficit, which may result in weight loss, by eating fewer calories and engaging in regular exercise.

Some people might decide to limit their daily caloric intake to 1,500. A 1,500-calorie intake is typically less than what the average person needs, even though caloric needs can vary depending on factors like age, gender, and level of activity. Therefore, this diet might aid in weight loss for some people.

We go over the 1,500-calorie diet's definition and safe practices in this Chapter.

**What is a diet of 1,500 calories?**

A person's daily calorie intake is capped at 1,500 calories under the 1,500-calorie diet. To regulate their eating and lose weight, people may try this diet.

Some claim that the typical female can lose 1 pound per week by keeping her daily caloric intake to 1,500 calories or less. To lose the same amount of weight, a typical male may eat up to 2,000 calories per day. However, other data suggest that there is significant individual variation in the amount of weight loss caused by a calorie deficit. As a result, the aforementioned guidelines should only be used as general guidelines.

The number of calories a person needs each day depends on a number of factors. These elements include age, gender, height, weight, and activity level.

One size fits all

Since everyone has different caloric needs, it is unlikely that any weight loss method will work for everyone.

1,500 calories a day as a goal may be too low for some people, making it unsustainable over time.

**Calories required**

The body receives the energy it requires to carry out its
functions from the calories found in food and beverages.
Eating too many calories can result in weight gain,
which may lead to obesity, and other medical conditions
like gout, breathing difficulties, heart disease, high blood
pressure, stroke, type 2 diabetes, gallstones, fertility
issues, and social and mental health problems.
A person's health can also be harmed by eating too little.
Anorexia and bulimia can be very dangerous because the
body cannot function properly on an extremely
restrictive diet.
Calorie requirements vary from person to person in order
to maintain bodily functions. The estimated daily caloric
requirements for adults are listed below, broken down by
age, gender, and level of activity.

Males

| Age | Sedentary | Moderate | Active |
| --- | --- | --- | --- |
| 19–20 | 2,600 | 2,800 | 3,000 |
| 21–25 | 2,400 | 2,800 | 3,000 |
| 26–35 | 2,400 | 2,600 | 3,000 |
| 36–40 | 2,400 | 2,600 | 2,800 |
| 41–45 | 2,200 | 2,600 | 2,800 |
| 46–55 | 2,200 | 2,400 | 2,800 |
| 56–60 | 2,200 | 2,400 | 2,600 |

| Age | Sedentary | Moderate | Active |
| --- | --- | --- | --- |
| 61–65 | 2,000 | 2,400 | 2,600 |
| 66–75 | 2,000 | 2,200 | 2,600 |
| 76 and up | 2,000 | 2,200 | 2,400 |

Females

| Age | Sedentary | Moderate | Active |
| --- | --- | --- | --- |
| 19–25 | 2,000 | 2,200 | 2,400 |
| 26–30 | 1,800 | 2,000 | 2,400 |
| 31–50 | 1,800 | 2,000 | 2,200 |
| 51–60 | 1,600 | 1,800 | 2,200 |
| 61 and up | 1,600 | 1,800 | 2,000 |

These calorie estimates do not account for values for expectant or nursing mothers.

A person must be aware of their daily energy expenditure in order to calculate how many calories they will need to maintain their bodily functions (TDDE). The TDEE is a calculation of a person's daily caloric requirements. People must consume fewer calories than the calculated amount in order to lose weight.

Minimum resting energy requirements are represented by the basal metabolic rate (BMR). The TDEE is also influenced by exercise. In order to determine BMR, nutritionists may:

• Males: 5 x age in years + 5 x weight in kilograms (kg) + 6.25 x height in centimeters (cm)

• Females: 10 times weight (kg) plus 6.25 times height (cm) minus 5 times age (years) – 161

People can use an online calculator to determine their BMR. People can use this calculator to determine their TDEE while also accounting for their level of physical activity.

**Foods to Consume**

A person may decide to eat nutrient-dense foods if their objective is to lose weight or maintain their health. The following foods are included in the list of diet recommendations:

• Vegetables in deep green, red, and orange hues.

• Cruciferous vegetables

Legumes, fruits, whole grains, enriched grains, dairy products without added fat or with reduced fat, lean meats, poultry, and eggs, as well as unsalted nuts, seeds, and soy products.

**Noxious Foods**

The recommendations make it clear to stay away from some foods. These include foods that have extra salt, sugar, or fat. Some people may find it challenging to adhere to extremely strict diets, so nutritionists may recommend: • limiting added sugar to less than 10% of daily calories

• keeping sodium intake below 2,300 milligrams per day; • keeping saturated fats to less than 10% of daily calories.

## GM DIET

There is a 7-day meal plan for the GM diet. Focus on a different food or food group every day. The GM diet encourages weight loss in a number of ways, such as:

 • By urging individuals to consume more fruit and vegetables, which are nutritious, low-calorie foods.

• forbids processed foods or added sugars

• reduces people's daily calorie intake and forbids refined carbohydrates

Due to the GM diet's emphasis on consuming fewer calories than one expends, dieters are likely to experience weight loss. It is unlikely to be the healthiest method of weight loss, though.

Because every person has a unique body, different people may have different experiences.

**What is the GM diet?**

On the GM diet, each day's meals consist of a different food group or combination of food groups. Fruits, vegetables, meat, and milk are the primary food groups permitted by the GM diet.

The strategy instructs people to eat a big breakfast, a reasonably sized lunch, and a light dinner. Additionally, it permits several snacks throughout the day.

The diet also calls for the consumption of "wonder soup," a tangy, low-calorie vegetable soup made with carrots, celery, tomatoes, and cabbage. Wonder soup can be consumed as a snack to stave off hunger until the next meal.

The program advises people to consume plenty of water in order to encourage healthy digestion and prevent fatigue. With each meal, the plan advises drinking 2-3 glasses of water. Depending on a person's age, body weight, and general health, there is no set amount of water that should be consumed every day.

Individuals behind the GM diet can take part in light forms of workout, such as yoga while dieting. After day 3, they can increase their cardio routine with walking or other low-intensity exercises. People can begin incorporating strength training into their exercise routine on days five through seven.

We outline the GM diet's fundamental components and offer sample meal plans below:

Day 1: Fruit

People can eat a choice of fruits, especially melons and citrus fruits, but should evade bananas.

A medium apple or a bowl of mixed berries for breakfast. A bowl of cantaloupe or an orange for a snack.

1 bowl of watermelon for lunch.

Snack: 1 bowl of mixed berries; dinner: 1 pear or 1 bowl of kiwi; dinner: 1 orange

Day 2: vegetables

Sweet potatoes or baked potatoes are good ways to start the day, but only have potatoes for breakfast. Vegetables can be consumed either raw or cooked.

• Snack: 1 bowl of cabbage; breakfast: 1 baked potato or 1 sweet potato

• A mixed salad with lettuce, tomatoes, carrots, and cucumber for lunch

Snack: 1 container of cucumber slices. Dinner: 1 bowl of kale or arugula with asparagus. Snack: 1 container of steamed or fresh broccoli.

Day 3: Vegetables and fruits

The same foods from days 1 and 2 may be consumed, with the exception of bananas and potatoes.

Lunch is a mixed salad; the snack is a bowl of sliced cucumbers. Breakfast consists of an apple or a bowl of watermelon.

• Snack: 1 apple; dinner: 1 kale salad with carrots, cucumbers, and 1 bowl of strawberries on the side

Day 4: Milk and bananas

Eat bananas whole or blend them with milk and ice to make a smoothie. No other fruits or vegetables are permitted, but wonder soup is available for consumption.

• Two bananas and a glass of milk for breakfast

• Snack: 1 smoothie made with skim milk and banana.

One bowl of wonder soup for lunch; one smoothie with banana and skim milk for a snack.

• Wonder soup and one banana for dinner

Day 5: Meat

20 ounces (oz) of beef, chicken, or fish should be consumed. Brown rice or cottage cheese can be used in place of meat for vegetarians.

• For breakfast, a serving of 5–6 ounces of meat and 2 whole tomatoes

The following are the details of the event.

• Four more cups of water

Day 6: Meat and vegetables

20 ounces of meat and as many cooked or raw vegetables as you want, but not potatoes or tomatoes.

Brown rice or cottage cheese can be substituted for meat for vegetarians.

• For breakfast, serve 1 bowl of vegetables and 5–6 ounces of meat.

• For lunch, have a 7-8 ounce serving of meat and a bowl of vegetables.

5-6 ounces of meat served with wonder soup for dinner; wonder soup for snacks.

Day 7: Vegetables, fruit, and rice

Consume brown rice, vegetables, and fruit. Juice without sugar is permitted as part of the diet for today.

Lunch consists of one bowl of brown rice and a glass of sugar-free fruit juice. Breakfast consists of one bowl of brown rice and an orange or bowl of watermelon.

Snacks include berries, citrus fruits, or wonder soup. Dinner consists of 1 bowl of brown rice and 1 bowl of raw or cooked vegetables.

**Benefits**

The GM diet has a number of related advantages and risks.

Additional fruits and vegetables

The following is a list of the items that are included in the package. Fruits and vegetables prevent the body from storing fat because they have few calories and a lot of fiber, which keeps people satisfied for longer.

Fewer sugars added

The GM diet prohibits the addition of sugar to any food or beverage, including alcohol.

Americans typically consume and drink more sugar than is healthy. I found associations between added sugar-rich diets and a number of diseases, such as obesity, heart disease, and type 2 diabetes.

The Centers for Disease Control and Avoidance (CDC) counsel individuals to consume no more than 10% of their day-to-day calories from added sugars.

Other advantages

Other impressive outcomes allegedly experienced by those who adhere to the GM diet include improved skin quality and appearance; improved mood; and improved digestion and metabolism.

• Detoxification

• treating IBS, constipation, and diarrhea

It's crucial to remember that there isn't enough evidence to back up these claims.

**Risks**

Although it might be alluring to think that you can lose a lot of weight quickly, there are risks associated with the GM diet.

**Lacking vital nutrients**

The GM diet may cause people to consume insufficient amounts of certain key food groups, such as protein and healthy fats. Additionally, their diet might be deficient in the important vitamins and minerals that come from consuming a variety of wholesome foods.

The body requires healthy unsaturated fats to function, even though Tran's fats, which are prevalent in many fried and baked foods, can raise cholesterol and have negative health effects.

Unsaturated fats, like those found in walnuts, avocados, and salmon, help lower cholesterol and have additional health advantages.

I contend that eating a lot of protein helps people lose weight and brings down their cholesterol and blood sugar levels. Such eating plans may also lessen feelings of hunger and boost metabolic function. The GM diet may not provide enough protein for some people.

**Loss of weight quickly**

The GM diet is not recommended as a long-term weight-loss plan, so once it is stopped, a person may gain the weight back.

This is due, in part, to the fact that the diet does not always impart the skills necessary for long-term weight maintenance, such as cooking and eating healthy foods.

Long-term lifestyle changes, such as increasing exercise and cooking with a variety of healthy ingredients, are more effective for maintaining weight loss than short-term diet plans.

Other dangers

One GM diet also lists the following risks: dehydration, muscle weakness, fatigue, headaches, and poor physical performance during exercise.

# CHAPTER 2

## UNDERSTANDING MACRONUTRIENTS

Macronutrients, also known as "macros," are nutrients that your body needs in large quantities to operate at its best. The three main macronutrients are carbs, protein, and fat.

Your body receives energy and the nutrients it needs to maintain its structure and functions from a group of nutrients known as macronutrients.

The term "macro" refers to their relative need for them being in greater quantities than other nutrients. Despite the fact that there are recommended ranges for macronutrient intake, your requirements depend on your unique situation.

This chapter discusses the primary macronutrients, food sources, uses, and how to determine your macronutrient requirements.

**What are macronutrients?**

Your body requires a lot of nutrients called macronutrients to operate at their best.

The three main macronutrients are fat, protein, and carbohydrates. They are regarded as essential nutrients, which means your body either cannot produce them or cannot produce them in sufficient amounts.

For instance, essential amino acids are provided by proteins, and essential fatty acids are present in fats. These elements are used by your body for certain purposes.

Calorie-based energy is also present in macronutrients. The majority of your body's energy comes from carbohydrates, but it can also draw on other macronutrients if necessary.

Each macronutrient contains 4 calories per gram of carbohydrate, 4 calories of protein, and 9 calories of fat. The nutrients that your body requires in large quantities are known as macronutrients and include fat, carbohydrates, and protein. They are often referred to as "macros" and are the nutrients that give you energy. The nutrients found in food that your body needs to maintain its systems and structures are found in macronutrients. All three macronutrients are necessary for a healthy diet, so you shouldn't seriously limit or exclude any of them.

**What Amount Of Protein Is Required?**

Protein is necessary for a number of bodily processes, including:

• The hormonal system; the metabolic system; the transport system; and the enzymes that control metabolism

• Keeping the acid/base environment in balance

Your protein requirements are influenced by your weight and level of exercise. A typical sedentary man needs about 56 grams of protein per day. The recommended daily intake for a sedentary woman is about 46 grams. You can safely eat more protein the more active you are. Aim for 10% to 35% of your daily calories to come from protein. Protein cannot be stored by the body. Your body will turn the remaining amount into energy or fat once you've reached the amount required. After meeting your daily calorie needs, concentrate on consuming carbohydrates and fat for the remaining calories.

**Carbohydrates Needed**

Your body uses carbohydrates as fuel when engaging in vigorous exercise. They enable your body to utilize carbohydrates rather than protein when you exercise, maintaining your muscle mass. Carbohydrates also give your central nervous system, which includes your brain, energy.

Your body uses carbohydrates as its main fuel source. Between 45% and 65% of your daily calories should come from carbohydrates. Similar to protein, the type of food from which you obtain your carbohydrates is crucial. Both healthy and unhealthy foods contain carbohydrates.

Carbohydrates from the healthiest sources can give you fiber, vitamins, minerals, and phytochemicals. Plants contain substances called phytochemicals that may be used to treat disease. These include whole grains, beans, vegetables, and fruits that have not been processed.

Your blood sugar may spike if you consume carbohydrates from unwholesome sources. They can cause diabetes, heart disease, and weight gain. Easy-to-digest foods like white bread, pastries, soda, and other highly processed foods are among them.

What Amount Of Fat Is Required?

Your diet should contain fat in moderation. Your body needs fat for the following reasons: absorbing fat-soluble vitamins, such as vitamins K, E, D, and A; insulating your body and protecting your organs; producing essential fatty acids that your body cannot make; serving as a component of cell walls; providing energy.

Try to get 20% to 35% of your daily caloric intake from fat. It's crucial to obtain your fat from healthy sources, just like you should with other macronutrients. The strongest types of fat come from plants and are called monounsaturated and polyunsaturated.

Since they are linked to high levels of bad cholesterol and internal inflammation, saturated fat, which is primarily found in animal sources and tropical oils, shouldn't make up more than 7% to 10% of your diet. Saturated fat comes from sources like beef, pork, lamb, veal, and high-fat dairy products.

Butter, processed baked goods like pastries, processed meat like hot dogs, and coconut and palm oil Trans-fat should be avoided because it raises your bad cholesterol while lowering your good cholesterol. Only products made from animals contain cholesterol. You should consume no more than 300 grams of cholesterol per day if your cholesterol levels are normal. If your cholesterol is high, keep your daily calorie intake to under 200 grams.

## FUNCTIONS OF MACRONUTRIENTS

Every macronutrient in your body serves a specific purpose.

They are divided into smaller pieces during digestion. These components are then utilized by the body for processes like cell division, cellular organization, and energy production.

Carbs

The majority of carbohydrates decompose into glucose or sugar molecules. Dietary fiber, a type of carbohydrate that isn't digested and moves through your body undigested, is an exception to this rule. Still, bacteria in your colon ferment some fiber.

Carbs serve a number of important purposes, including

• Instant energy. Your brain, central nervous system, and red blood cells prefer glucose as an energy source.

• Energy storage. Glycogen, a form of glucose that is stored in your muscles and liver for use when you need energy, such as after a prolonged fast, is released when you need it.

• Digestion. Fiber helps maintain regular bowel movements.

• Aids in promoting satiety. After eating, fiber fills you up and prolongs your feeling of fullness.

Proteins

Amino acids are formed during protein digestion. Nine of the twenty amino acids, which are essential and must be obtained from food, play significant roles in your body.

Amino acids from proteins are primarily used for repairing and building. Your body uses amino acids to make new proteins. Additionally, they help to develop and restore muscles and tissues.

• Giving direction. Your body's cell membranes, organs, hair, skin, and nails all have structure thanks to amino acids.

• pH harmony. Your body's proper acid-base balance is supported by amino acids.

• Producing hormones and enzymes. Your body cannot produce enzymes and hormones without the proper amino acids.

Fats

Fatty acids and glycerol are formed when fats are broken down.

Lipids, also known as fats, are essential for maintaining the health of cell membranes. A vital part of cell membranes is lipids.

• Energy storage. When you eat fewer calories than you burn, the fat that is stored throughout your body can be used as an energy reserve.

• Absorption and transportation. The fat-soluble vitamins K, E, D, and A are supported in their transport and absorption by lipids.

• Insulation. Your organs are protected and insulated by fat.

## COMPARING MACRONUTRIENTS AND MICRONUTRIENTS

Macronutrients are different from micronutrients, which include vitamins and minerals.

First, compared to micronutrients, macronutrients are required in relatively higher amounts. Micronutrients are still important, despite this fact.

In your body, macronutrients play one set of roles while micronutrients play another. Each essential vitamin and mineral has a distinct, occasionally overlapping function. There are 13 essential vitamins and minerals.

Remind yourself that essentially means you must obtain those nutrients from your diet. Your body is capable of producing some vitamins—including biotin, D, K, and B12—but not always in sufficient quantities. Micronutrients support growth, brain development, immune function, and energy metabolism.

Micronutrients don't have calories, but macronutrients do because they are the building blocks of your body's structure and functions. Instead, they are essential for converting food into energy and facilitating the majority of bodily functions.

Large amounts of macronutrients are necessary for your body to function. Micronutrients are necessary for very small amounts for your body to function properly. The micronutrients are.

Vitamins that are water-soluble. Folic acid, vitamin C, vitamin B1, vitamin B2, vitamin B6, and vitamin B12 are some of these vitamins.

The vitamin that is fat-soluble. These include vitamins A, D, E, and K, which can be found in foods that contain fat.

**Minerals.**

 All minerals are micronutrients, but some minerals are more essential to your body than others. All the minerals your body requires are typically provided by a balanced diet. Macro minerals are those that your body requires more of and include: sodium, chloride, potassium, calcium, phosphorus, magnesium, and sulfur.

Micro minerals or trace minerals are minerals that your body doesn't require as much of and include:

• Iron

- Zinc
- Iodine
- Selenium
- Copper
- Manganese
- Fluoride
- Chromium
- Molybdenum

In very small amounts, your body also requires certain minerals. These are: Nickel, Silicon, Vanadium, Cobalt, and

**Macro Analysis to Use**

Every macronutrient is crucial for your body to function at its best. It's essential to consume enough protein, fat, and carbohydrates by following a balanced diet that includes a variety of foods.

These Acceptable Macronutrient Distribution Ranges (AMDR) for adults are recommended by the United States Department of Agriculture's (USDA) Dietary Guidelines:

- Carbs account for 45-65% of your daily calories.

- Protein makes up 10 to 35% of your daily calories.

- Fat makes up 20–35% of your daily calories.

The recommendations state that adults should consume at least 130 grams of carbohydrates each day. This is the Recommended Dietary Allowance (RDA), which is thought to be the minimum amount required to give your brain enough glucose.

Your body can get energy from breaking down fat and protein if there isn't enough glucose available, which can happen if you're strictly following a ketogenic diet or have trouble controlling your insulin levels because of conditions like diabetes.

Adults need at least 0.36 grams of protein per pound (0.8 grams per kilogram) of body weight.

But remember that each person's required intake of macronutrients differs depending on their age, level of activity, sex, and other factors.

For proper brain development, for instance, children and adolescents may require more fat-containing calories than adults.

On the other hand, older adults require more protein to maintain muscle mass. Numerous specialists endorse a protein intake of at least 0.45-0.54 grams per pound (1.0-1.2 grams per kg) for adults over the age of 65.

They should aim for the higher end of the recommended ranges as athletes and people who are highly active frequently need more carbs and protein than people who are less active. Extra protein helps rebuild muscles after exercise, while carbs give you calories to refuel your energy.

You may benefit from eating slightly fewer calories from carbohydrates and more calories from protein if you're trying to lose weight. Fewer carbs can encourage a calorie deficit, while more protein can make you feel more satisfied.

**Do you really need to count macros?**

Counting macros is a weight loss strategy that is becoming more and more popular. This tactic is also used by some athletes or people who need a certain amount of a macronutrient, like protein for building muscle.

Planning your meals in accordance with your goal percentage of calories from each macronutrient group is typically required.

While macro counting can be a useful strategy for some individuals to achieve their objectives, it is not required for everyone. In fact, if you consume sources of each macronutrient in a well-balanced diet, you probably meet the recommended intake.

One easy way to make sure you eat enough carbohydrates, proteins, and fats is to simply put together a balanced plate at each meal.

As a general rule, half of your plate should be non-starchy vegetables, a quarter should be high-fiber carbs, such as fruit or whole grains, and a quarter should be a source of protein. Make using healthy fats a priority when cooking.

Consider working with a registered dietitian to identify and meet your needs if you're interested in assessing your macronutrient intake further.

Never forget that meeting a certain amount every day is not as important as the quality of the macronutrients in your diet.

For instance, you won't get nearly as many nutrients and fiber from eating sugary treats and refined carbohydrates to meet your daily carb goal as you would from eating fruits, vegetables, and whole grains.

## FOOD SOURCES FOR FAT, PROTEIN, AND CARBOHYDRATES

The foods you eat can provide macronutrients for you. To consume enough of each macronutrient, a variety of foods should be consumed.
Most foods are a mixture of fat, protein, and carbohydrates.
Some foods have a high concentration of a single macronutrient, while others have high concentrations of two nutrients and belong to two different macronutrient groups.
Carbohydrate sources include:
• Whole grains, including barley, faro, oats, and brown rice
Peas, potatoes, corn, and other starchy vegetables are among the vegetables.
• Fruits, including figs, apples, mangoes, and bananas

Black beans, lentils, and chickpeas are among the legumes. Milk and yogurt are dairy products.

Among the sources of protein are:

• Poultry, particularly chicken, and turkey;
• Eggs, especially egg whites
• Seafood: salmon, shrimp, and cod; and red meat: beef, lamb, and pork
• Dairy products, such as cheese, yogurt, and milk
• Legumes and beans, including chickpeas, lentils, and black beans
• Seeds and nuts, such as pumpkin seeds and almonds
• Tofu, edamame, and tempeh are products made from soy.

These are some sources of fat:

• Extra virgin olive oil
• Fresh, dried, and coconut oil from the coconut
• Fresh avocados and avocado oil
• Seeds and nuts, such as pumpkin seeds and almonds
• Oily fish, such as herring and salmon
• Dairy products: cheese and yogurt with added fat.

# CHAPTER 3

## EATING FOR MAXIMUM HEALTH

Start small when trying to eat healthier. Try to avoid processed foods and include nutrient-dense foods in each meal and snack.

Depending on whom you ask, "healthy eating" may take many forms. Everyone seems to have an opinion on the healthiest diet, including medical professionals, wellness influencers, coworkers, and family members.

Additionally, online nutrition items can be extremely perplexing due to their contradictory — and frequently erroneous — advice and guidelines.

If all you want to do is eat in a way that is healthy for you, this makes it difficult.

The truth is that eating a healthy diet doesn't have to be difficult. It is entirely possible to eat the foods you love and still nourish your body.

Food should not be feared, counted, weighed, or tracked; rather, it should be enjoyed.

**Important Of Healthy Eating**

It's important to first discuss why healthy eating matters before delving further into what it entails.

First and foremost, food provides you with the energy and nutrients your body needs to function. Your well-being may hurt if your diet is low in calories or one or more nutrients.

Similarly to this, consuming too many calories can result in weight gain. Obese individuals are much more likely to develop conditions like type 2 diabetes, obstructive sleep apnea, and heart, liver, and kidney disease.

Your diet's quality also has an impact on your risk of contracting diseases, longevity, and mental health.

Diets consisting primarily of whole, nutrient-dense foods are linked to increased longevity and disease protection, whereas diets high in ultra-processed foods are linked to increased mortality and a higher risk of conditions like cancer and heart disease.

Highly processed food-rich diets may also increase the risk of depressive symptoms, especially in those who exercise less frequently.

Additionally, if your current diet is heavy on ultra-processed items like fast food, soda, and sugary cereals but light on whole foods like vegetables, nuts, and fish, you're probably not getting enough of some nutrients, which could have a negative impact on your general health.

**Does eating healthfully require adhering to a specific diet?**

Without a doubt!

Utmost individuals don't need to obey to any specific diet in order to feel their best, even though some individuals need to avoid certain foods or accept diets for health reasons.

That is not to say that you cannot benefit from some eating habits.

For instance, some people find that a low-carb diet makes them feel the healthiest, while high-carb diets suit other people better.

However, generally speaking, eating healthily has nothing to do with following a diet or specific dietary guidelines. Simply put, "healthy eating" refers to putting your health first by nourishing your body with wholesome foods.

Depending on each person's location, financial situation, culture, society, and taste preferences, the specifics may vary.

## FUNDAMENTAL ELEMENTS OF A HEALTHY DIET

Now that you are conscious of the remunerations of eating well, let's discuss some basics of nutrition.

**Nutrient content**

Your first thought when thinking about healthy eating may be related to calories. Although calories are significant, nutrients should be your top priority.

The term "nutrient density" describes the ratio of a food's nutrient content to its caloric content.

While calories are existing in all foods, not all foods are nutrient-dense.

For example, while a candy bar or a box of mac and cheese may have a ration of calories, they don't cover any vitamins, minerals, protein, or fiber. Likewise, foods labeled "diet-friendly" or "low calorie" may contain very few calories but be deficient in nutrients.

For instance, compared to whole eggs, egg whites have significantly fewer calories and fat. However, a whole egg contains 5-21% of the Daily Value (DV) for the nutrients iron, phosphorus, zinc, choline, and vitamins A and B12, whereas an egg white only offers 1% or less of the DV.

That is a result of the egg's healthy, high-fat yolk. Additionally, while many foods that are high in nutrients, such as a variety of fruits and vegetables, are low in calories, others, such as nuts, full-fat dairy products, egg yolks, avocados, and fatty fish, are often high in calories. That's totally fine!

Likewise, food doesn't automatically qualify as a healthy option just because it has few calories.

You're missing the point of healthy eating if all of your food decisions are made solely on the basis of calories. Try to eat a common of foods that are high in vitamins, minerals, fiber, healthy fats, and nutrients like protein.

**Dietary variety**

Dietary diversity, or consuming a variety of foods, is another aspect of healthy eating.

A diet full of a variety of foods supports your gut flora, encourages a healthy body weight, and guards against chronic disease.

Still, if you're a picky eater, it might be challenging to eat a variety of foods.

Try presenting fresh foods one at a time if that's the case. If you don't consume many vegetables, start by including a favorite vegetable in one or two meals each day, and then increase your intake from there.

Despite the fact that you might not enjoy trying new foods, research demonstrates that the more exposure you have a food, the higher the possibility that you will develop adapted to it.

**Ratios of macronutrients**

Carbs, fat, and protein are macronutrients, or the primary nutrients you obtain from food. (Fiber is observed as a kind of carb.)

Mostly speaking, you should stabilize the three during your meals and snacks. Particularly, making dishes rich in fiber more filling and delicious by incorporating protein and fat.

When you nosh on fruit, for example, joining it with a spoonful of nut butter or a small amount of cheese aids you feel fuller longer than if you were to eat the fruit alone.

However, it's okay if your diet isn't consistently balanced.

Most individuals don't need to count macros or follow to a rigid macronutrient plan, with the omission of athletes, those trying to attain a definite body structure, and those who must increase their muscle mass or body fat for health aims.

Additionally, obsessing over maintaining a specific macro range and counting macros can result in disordered eating behaviors or a harmful fixation on food and calories.

It's important to keep in mind that some people may do well on diets that are high in fat and protein, low in carbs, or low in fat and high in carbs. However, it's not usually necessary to count macronutrients on these diets either.

For instance, choosing low-carb foods like no starchy vegetables, proteins, and fats more frequently than high-carb foods will classically be adequate if you feel your best on a low-carb diet.

**High levels of processing**

Reducing your intake of highly processed foods is one of the best ways to improve your diet.

You are not required to completely avoid processed foods. In actuality, a lot of wholesome foods have undergone some form of processing, including shelled nuts, canned beans, and frozen fruits and vegetables.

Contrarily, heavily processed foods like soda, commercially baked goods, candy, sugary cereals, and some boxed snacks contain little to no whole-food ingredients.

High fructose corn syrup, hydrogenated oils, and artificial sweeteners are frequently found in these products.

Study relative's diets high in ultra-processed foods to a bigger risk of misery, heart disease, obesity, and many other difficulties.

Conversely, diets high in whole, nutrient-dense foods and low in these foods have the opposite effect, extending lifespan, preventing disease, and enhancing overall physical and mental well-being.

So it is best to prioritize nutrient-dense foods, especially fruits, and vegetables.

Should you limit certain foods and drinks for the best health?

It's best to limit certain foods in a healthy diet.

Ultra-processed foods are associated with poor health outcomes, such as an increased risk of disease and early death, according to decades of scientific research.

Reducing your consumption of highly processed packaged snacks, soda, processed meats, candy, ice cream, fried foods, and fast food is a wise move that will improve your health and lower your risk of developing certain diseases.

You don't have to always completely avoid these foods, though.

Save highly processed foods and beverages for special occasions and try to prioritize whole, nutrient-dense foods like vegetables, fruits, nuts, seeds, beans, and fish. Ice cream and candy can be included in a balanced, healthy diet, but they shouldn't make up a large portion of your daily caloric intake.

## HOW TO FAMILIARIZE A HEALTHY DIET TO YOUR LIFE

One of the many pieces that make up your daily life is food. Food may be the least of your daily worries after commuting, working, having family or social obligations, running errands, and many other things. Making food a priority is the first step to maintaining a healthier diet.

This doesn't mean that you have to spend hours making elaborate meals or meal prepping, but it does mean that you need to put some thought and effort into it, especially if you lead a very busy lifestyle.

For instance, making sure you shop for groceries once or twice a week will help you make sure your fridge and pantry are stocked with healthy options. Consequently, having a fully stocked kitchen makes it much simpler to select healthy meals and snacks.

Stock up on fresh and frozen produce, protein sources like chicken, eggs, fish, and tofu, bulk carbs like canned beans and whole grains, starchy vegetables like potatoes,

butternut squash, and white and sweet potatoes, and fat sources like avocados, olive oil, and full-fat yogurt when you go grocery shopping.
• Wholesome, easy-to-prepare snack foods like nuts, seeds, nut butter, hummus, olives, and dried fruit
When you're at the table and sense stuck, keep it forthright and think in threes:
Suitable sources of fat include olive oil, nuts, seeds, nut butter, avocado, cheese, and full-fat yogurt. Suitable sources of protein include eggs, chicken, fish, or tofu.
• Fiber-rich carbohydrates include starchy foods like sweet potatoes, oats, some fruits, and beans as well as low-carb options like berries, asparagus, broccoli, and cauliflower.
For instance, a lunchtime sweet potato stuffed with vegetables, beans, and shredded chicken, and a dinnertime salmon filet or baked tofu with sautéed broccoli and brown rice might be options for breakfast. Focus on one meal if you're not used to cooking or grocery shopping. Buy the ingredients for a few breakfast or dinner dishes for the forthcoming week at the grocery store. Once that is fixed in your routine, add more meals until you are cooking utmost of them yourself.
It might take some time to establish a positive relationship with food.
You're not alone if you don't have a positive relationship with food.
Eating conditions or propensities toward disordered eating are common. It's crucial to get the appropriate help if you have concerns that you may have one of these conditions.

You require the appropriate equipment if you want to form a positive affiliation with food.

The best way to begin repairing your relationship with food is to work with a healthcare side, such as a enumerated dietitian and psychologist who focusses in eating disorders.

Food restrictions, fad diets, and self-diagnosed ideas like "getting back on track" won't help and might even be detrimental. It might take some time, but improving your relationship with food is essential for both your physical and mental health.

## ADVICE FOR EATING WELL IN THE REAL WORLD

Here are specific useful ideas to help you start eating healthily:

• Give plant-based foods a top priority. Your diet should be primarily composed of plant foods like fruits, vegetables, beans, and nuts. Consider including these foods, particularly fruits, and vegetables, at each meal and snack.

Cook meals at home. Having a diverse diet is made stress-free by cooking at home. If you're used to eating out or ordering takeout, start by cooking only one or two meals per week.

• Regular grocery shopping. You're more likely to prepare healthy meals and snacks if your kitchen is stocked with healthy foods. Make one or two daily grocery rounds to ensure you have a source of healthy foods.

• Diagnose that your diet won't be faultless. Develop, not rightness, is what matters. Wherever you are, accept yourself. Cooking one homemade, nutrient-dense meal per week if you currently eat out every night is a significant improvement.

• "Cheat days" are not allowed. Having "cheat days" or "cheat meals" on a consistent basis specifies that your diet is out of stability. There is no need to cheat once you realize that all foods can be a part of a healthy diet.

• Avoid sugar-sweetened beverages. As much as you can, shun drinking sugary beverages like soda, vitality drinks, and sweet coffee. Drinking sugary beverages regularly can be bad for your health.

• Opt for filling meals. When you're starving, you should aim to eat adequately, healthy foods rather than trying to consume as few calories as likely. Choose meals and snacks that are high in protein and fiber to keep you full.

• Consume whole foods. Whole foods like vegetables, fruits, beans, nuts, seeds, whole grains, and protein sources like eggs and fish should make up the majority of a healthy diet.

• Drink water carefully. Healthy eating includes staying hydrated, and the best way to do so is with water. Get a reusable water bottle and flavor it with fruit slices or a squeeze of lemon if you're not used to drinking water.

• Respect your distastes. Don't eat something if you've tried it several times and don't like it. There are lots of nourishing foods obtainable as replacements. Just because something is regarded as healthy doesn't mean you have to eat it.

You can move toward a healthier diet by using these suggestions.

If you're unsure of where to begin when it comes to improving your diet, you can also consult a registered dietitian. A dietitian can assist you in creating an attainable, wholesome eating strategy that suits your needs and schedule.

# CHAPTER 4

## GROCERY SHOPPING AND MEAL PLANNING

**M**eal planning doesn't have to be challenging or time-consuming. I have been using this easy meal-planning technique every week for years. For this busy mother, it makes choosing meals and going grocery shopping much faster and simpler!

I frequently get asked to describe my meal planning process, so even though I frequently give sneak peeks, I thought it would be useful to have everything outlined in one place on the blog. Although I've used other techniques in the past, the steps I outlined in this post are the ones I've faithfully followed for a few years (at least).

I'm not telling you that this should be your process when I walk you through mine. Meal planning doesn't really have a one-size-fits-all method. However, I firmly believe that there are methods and strategies that most people can adapt and use to make meal planning simpler.

Every weekend I take out my bullet journal (more on that here), and I turn to the page where I keep track of my meals. I remove the previous week's post-it and replace it with a new one before following the instructions. The process is incredibly easy because I follow the same steps every week and have everything I need (master lists, shopping lists, and a meal plan) in one place. The process that takes the longest is probably asking my husband about his weekly schedule.

Anyone interested in simple meal planning can use the general steps I outline below. I provide more information about how I complete each step, along with links to other resources you might find helpful, under each step. I'm hoping these pointers will help you in the future make meal planning a little simpler. Just keep in mind that it might take some time to really find your groove and that sometimes putting in a little effort upfront (like making a master list) can save you a lot of time and effort down the road.

**Write down everything we already have as a first step.**

I quickly complete this each week using my Kitchen Essentials Checklist. I used to print off a copy every week, but about a year ago, I had the brilliant idea to laminate it and keep it in my bullet journal next to my meal planning page. This simple action completely transformed my life. For your printing convenience, I've provided essential lists that are both filled in and empty.

I have three dry-erase markers on hand just for this step. I use my black marker to mark what we have, and then my red or orange marker to indicate what we are missing (red for items we get from Whole Foods, and orange for items we get at Costco).

When I'm at the store, this color-coded system will serve as my grocery list. It only takes one easy step and serves two purposes.

**Write down upcoming events or unique circumstances as the second step.**

The next thing I do after making a list of what we have on hand is to make a note of any events during the week that might have an impact on our various meals. A mini-conference with my husband is also necessary to ensure that there are no "surprises" during the week.

Days when we will be out of the house for the majority of the day and an easy dinner would be useful; days when my husband won't be home for dinner and it'll just be me and the kids; nights we have extra-curricular out of the house (rare these days) and we need an "on the road dinner" or something waiting for us when we get home; meals that can be made ahead of time;

**Use master lists and short lists to choose meals in the third step.**

The process of choosing meals for your meal plan is greatly simplified by the restriction of a list of recipes you already know you enjoy and trust, even with all the options available in cookbooks on the shelf, recipes, and search results in Google.

Depending on the season (both figuratively and literally), I have a number of different lists I can consult. In my bullet journal, I also keep master lists for dinner and lunch, where I have written out the recipes for our go-to meals as well as those from my cookbook for quick access.

In addition to the more inclusive master lists, I also find using summarized, more specific lists useful for finding meals within confident factors. For instance, I currently base a lot of my lunch planning decisions on my Summer Lunch Menu. On nights when my husband is away, I frequently consult my Easy Dinners List for meal inspiration. (I printed both of them at 50% size and inserted them next to my meal plan page in my bullet journal.)

In order to replace it each week, I list the meals for the coming week on a post-it note in my bullet journal (see image above). I schedule my meals for lunch and dinner because it suits me well. Because I choose my meals based on what is happening each weekday, I also like to choose days in advance.

Of course, it also works if you'd prefer to make a list of potential meals for the week and decide later what order you'll eat them in. This is what I used to do when our weekdays appeared more routine. In order to use up leftovers before returning to the store for fresh groceries, I also always plan for leftovers for Saturday lunch. Don't forget to include on your shopping list any additional ingredients required for the meals you chose.

Free Meal Lists:

• A Massive List of Simple Dinner Options.

• 75+ Cheap Dinner Options

• Menu for Summer Lunch

• PRINTABLE OPTION for the Master Lunch List

• Totally Awesome List of Nutritious Snack Ideas.

• Resources & 50+ Fresh Summer Vegetable Recipes

• A nutritious grab-and-go picnic idea

**Fourth Step: Shop and, if you can prepare in advance.**

I do my weekly shopping at Whole Foods and Costco. The majority of the time, I go to Costco in person and have Whole Foods deliver my groceries. I value the simplicity and regularity of buying 95% of our groceries from just two stores at this time in my life. I don't have the time or energy to visit numerous stores in a single day or over the course of a week.

When I get home from the store, I put the groceries away and consider what I can prepare now to make later in the week's mealtimes simpler. This might involve browning meat, cooking a whole chicken, chopping vegetables, washing fruit, using an Instant Pot to cook beans, preparing salad dressings, etc.

**Fifth Step: Use the meal plan to meet your needs and those of your family. Serve the meal plan sparingly.**

Meal planning helps me make sure we have the ingredients we need for the week in the house, and it's also a HUGE gift to my future self to not have to decide what to eat during the week when the days are so busy and packed.

But if we have to abandon the plan one day (or two) or three days in a row due to unforeseen circumstances or simply because we feel like having a different meal than what is on the list, I don't feel the slightest bit guilty about it.

I frequently fail to complete everything on my list in a given week. When this occurs, I typically simply carry over any leftovers into the following week.

# CHAPTER 5

## EXERCISE AND FITNESS

The single most crucial thing you can do for your health is to exercise frequently, ideally every day. Exercise helps to improve mood, regulate appetite, and get a better night's sleep in the short term. It lowers the risk of dementia, depression, diabetes, heart disease, and many types of cancer over the long term. Why is exercise so crucial for older people?

It's a great time to start an exercise and fitness routine, whether you were physically active in the past or have never done so. Seniors need to maintain their physical fitness just as much as younger people do.

Why is exercise crucial for seniors? Virtually every system in your body benefits when your heart rate is elevated and your muscles are being worked, which enhances both your physical and mental health in numerous ways. Physical activity improves blood sugar control, lowers inflammation, strengthens bones, and prevents the development of dangerous plaque in the arteries. It also helps maintain healthy blood pressure and fights depression. A regular exercise regimen can also improve your sexual life, result in better-quality sleep, lower your risk of developing some cancers, and extend your life.

Because they are unsure of the kinds of exercise and fitness that are efficient and safe, as well as the appropriate amount of exercise, many older adults are reluctant to start moving. The good news is that any form of exercise is preferable to inactivity, so there's no harm in beginning slowly and building up to longer workouts. Your impartial should be at least 150 minutes of moderate-intensity workout per week, but if you can't start there, work your way up to that amount. Although there are a lot of exact adult fitness and exercise activities, you should also be physically active throughout the day by using the stairs, working in the yard, and playing with your grandchildren.

The common of elders who are involved in exercise and fitness can start without seeing a doctor, but there are some exclusions. Consult your doctor first if you have a serious medical condition like diabetes, high blood pressure, heart or lung disease, osteoporosis, or a neurological disorder. Get advice from your doctor if you have mobility issues like arthritis or poor balance.

**What form of exercise are the Best**

Although there are countless ways to exercise, specialists divide the physical activity into four broad classes based on what each requires of your body and how it helps you.

A higher heart rate is a sign of aerobic exercise. Although the majority of aerobic exercises involve moving your entire body, the heart and lungs receive the majority of attention (aerobic exercise is frequently referred to as "cardio" because it strengthens and benefits your cardiovascular system). If accomplished with sufficient strength, sports like walking, swimming, dancing, and cycling cause your heart to beat more speedily. Exercises that burn fat also raise mood, lessen inflammation, and normalize blood sugar.

Two to three times per week should be set aside for strength training, also referred to as resistance training. Exercises like squats, lunges, push-ups, and those done with resistance bands, weights, or machines help maintain and even increase muscle mass and strength. Firming muscles also strengthens bones, controls blood sugar, and increases balance, all of which support in preventing falls. Exercises that are both isometric and isotonic should be join together. Planks and holding leg lifts are instances of isometric exercises, which are done without moving. They are fantastic at preserving strength and enhancing stability. With isotonic exercises, you must maintain weight bearing throughout a range of motion. Stretching exercises keep your muscles and tendons elastic, reserve your posture, and develop mobility, especially as you age. Every day stretching can be done.

Exercises for balance make use of the various systems, including those of the inner ear, vision, muscles, and joints, that keep you upright and oriented. Yoga and tai chi are excellent balance exercises that can help you stay independent well into your senior years and prevent falls.

**Do I need to exercise a lot?**
Your current level of fitness, your fitness objectives, the types of exercise you plan to do, and whether you have shortages in areas like strength, flexibility, or stability will all impact how much exercise you should be attaining.

Generally speaking, a weekly minimum of 150 minutes of moderate-intensity aerobic activity (or 75 minutes of vigorous exercise) is advised. To get the most benefit as you get fitter, you should go beyond that. You can naturally divide the 150 minutes into five 30-minute sessions per week or into two 15-minute sessions spread out over the course of one day. Select a plan that works for your daily life.

Target to work all of your main muscle sets twice to three times per week during strength exercises, with a recovery period of 48 hours in between each session. Doing "total-body" exercises requires two weekly sessions. It will take more frequent workouts if you choose to divide your sessions into separate sessions to target different muscle groups (such as "leg day"). Just be sure to give yourself 48 hours of rest before working out a major muscle again.

Ask your doctor for advice on balance-specific exercises if you've noticed issues with your balance, such as unsteadiness, vertigo, or dizziness. Add three half-hour exercise and at least two 30-minute walks to your weekly plan.

It's best to stretch after a brief period of warming up or to do stretching exercises after your workout is finished. Expand each muscle set slowly and steadily, then release and repeat.

But what level of work out is extreme? After working out, you should anticipate some muscle soreness, especially at first. However, you may be overtraining if you notice that your body is simply not recovering between workouts. Keep in mind that older people require more recuperation time than younger people.

 An exercise program should make you feel good, with the exception of "welcome" muscle soreness. It's a good idea to have a backup plan in case something goes wrong. That doesn't mean you should stop exercising; it just means you should reduce the intensity or frequency of your workouts until you find the "sweet spot" where your body has been sufficiently "tired out" while still being sufficiently restored to attack your subsequent session with enthusiasm.

## ADVANTAGES OF EXERCISE

Your body and mind will benefit greatly from a well-planned exercise program.

Work out has been revealed to have affirmative effects on mental health. For example, a significant study discovered that sedentary people have a 44% higher risk of depression. Another reading start that exercising for 90 minutes a week, individuals with mild to adequate depression could attain outcomes similar to those brought on by antidepressants. Serotonin and dopamine, two brain chemicals that improve mood and reduce stress, appear to be the key.

We are all aware of how exercise can improve cardiovascular health. But how does physical activity decrease blood pressure? It's interesting to note that by making your circulatory system work harder during aerobic exercise, you temporarily raise your blood pressure. Nevertheless, after you stop exercising, your blood pressure proceeds to its previous level.

Although diet is also very important, a lot of people believe that exercise is a crucial component of weight loss, and they are not mistaken. What activity, however, Cardio exercises are excellent for burning calories and shedding fat in general. However, you shouldn't discount the benefits of strength training, which optimizes your body's lean muscle-to-fat ratio (it's also the best exercise for bone strength). When it comes to the one perfect exercise for weight loss, there is no Holy Grail. The exercise you'll perform consistently is the one to lose weight with. Exercise that will help you lose weight is anything that gets your heart rate up and gets your body moving while you're having fun and staying motivated. Even those who have severe limitations can and should engage in some form of physical activity. Senior-specific exercises have been created by experts that are low-impact, secure, and, if necessary, can be performed while sitting down.

Balance exercises for seniors can be performed while holding onto a chair or doorframe if you're worried about your risk of falling. You could, for instance, tighten your abdominal muscles while standing behind a chair and lifting one leg up to the level of the middle of the other leg's calf. As you advance, you might experiment with holding the chair with just one hand before letting go completely.

Seniors with limited abilities can still benefit from core-strengthening exercises. For instance, to perform a standard plank, hold yourself parallel to the floor, only letting your forearms and toes touch the mat. In a simpler variation, you can also rest your knees on the mat. The plank can also be performed while standing and leaning forward. You rest on the balls of your feet with your back straight, your elbows and forearms on a desk, table, or wall.

There are a change of elongating exercises for elders to suit individuals of different capacities. Try a full-body bounce in which you lie on your back, straighten your legs, and spread your hands along the floor past your head if holding poses on your hands and knees is impossible. Some stretches, like neck rotations and overhead stretches, can be performed while seated.

In actuality, sitting still allows you to perform a variety of exercises. Other chair workouts for elders include bicep curls, above dumbbell presses, shoulder blade squeezes, calf raises, sit-to-stands (chair squats), and knee extensions.

What cardiovascular exercises are recommended?

In order to strengthen your entire body, increase your endurance, and ensure your long-term health, the best exercise program will combine both aerobic and strength training. The best way to get the most out of your money is to invest it wisely. Cardio workouts are bigger when it comes to pulling down blood pressure, sustaining the health of your veins' inner walls, discharging enzymes that melt blood clots, and even inspiring the progress of new arteries feeding the heart. While strength training certainly has cardiovascular benefits.

The risk of type 2 diabetes is significantly reduced by regular aerobic exercise. Lower risk of diabetes also lowers the risk of heart disease because high blood sugar damages blood vessels and the anxieties that control the heart, even though it's not normally thought of as a heart problem. Exercise stimulates your body's cells to remove glucose (sugar) from the blood, which they do by developing increased sensitivity to insulin, a hormone essential for the metabolism of glucose. Exercise that helps you lose weight, especially in the midsection, will also help you avoid developing diabetes since obesity is a significant risk factor for the disease.

You already know that exercise is healthy for you, but how healthy? Learn how exercise can enhance your life, from mood-boosting to improving your sex life.

Want to feel better, be more energetic, and possibly live longer? Just get moving.

Regular physical activity and exercise have many positive health effects that are difficult to deny. Everyone, regardless of age, sex, or physical ability, benefits from exercise.

## WAYS THAT EXERCISING CAN MAKE YOU HAPPIER AND HEALTHIER.

**`1. Exercise reduces weight**

Exercise can help maintain weight loss or prevent excessive weight gain. Calorie burn occurs during physical activity. You burn more calories when you engage in more vigorous exercise.

Regular gym visits are great but don't stress if you can't find a significant amount of time to work out every day. Anything you do is preferable to doing nothing at all. Simply increase your daily activity to reap the benefits of exercise. Take the stairs instead of the elevator or work harder at your housework. The key is consistency.

**2. Exercise fights illnesses and conditions**

Is heart disease giving you pause? Want to lower your blood pressure? Whatever your current weight, exercising increases the "good" cholesterol known as high-density lipoprotein (HDL), and lowers the bad cholesterol known as triglycerides. Your blood continues to flow normally as a result of these two factors, lowering your risk of cardiovascular diseases.

Numerous health issues and concerns, such as stroke, metabolic syndrome, high blood pressure, type 2 diabetes, depression, anxiety, many types of cancer, arthritis, and falls, can be prevented or managed with regular exercise.

Additionally, it can help with cognitive development and reduce the risk of dying from any cause.

**3. Exercise lifts one's spirits**

Need some emotional support? Or do you need to unwind after a demanding day? Exercise in the gym or a brisk walk can help. Different brain chemicals are stimulated by physical activity, which may make you feel happier, more at ease, and less anxious.

Regular exercise can also help you feel better about your appearance and yourself, which can increase your confidence and self-esteem.

4. Exercise increases energy Tired from household chores or grocery shopping? Your muscle strength and endurance can both increase with regular exercise. Exercise helps your cardiovascular system function more effectively and delivers oxygen and nutrients to your tissues. Additionally, you have more energy to complete daily tasks as your heart and lung health improves.

5. Workout helps you sleep well

Stressed to fall asleep? You can sleep well, deeper, and fall asleep more rapidly if you work out often. Just remember to avoid exercising right before bedtime if you don't want to be too energized to sleep.

**6. Exercise revitalizes your sexual life.**

Do you feel too worn out or unfit to enjoy intimate physical contact? Regular exercise can increase your energy levels and confidence in your physical appearance, which could enhance your sex life.
But there's even further to it than that. Steady workout may develop stimulation in women. Additionally, men who regularly exercise are less likely than men who don't to experience erectile dysfunction issues.

**7. working out can be enjoyable and social!**
Physical action and exercise can be pleasant. They give you the chance to relax, take in the outdoors, or just do things that make you happy. Additionally, engaging in physical activity can facilitate social interactions with loved ones or close friends.
So join a soccer team, go hiking, or take a dance class. Find a physical action you like, and just do it. Try something new or involve in activities with loved ones or friends.

**The Verdict on Exercise**
Physical activity and exercise are fantastic ways to feel better, improve your health, and have fun. The U.S. Department of Health and Human Services suggests the following exercise recommendations for the majority of healthy adults:
• Aerobic exercise. Get 75 minutes of vigorous aerobic exercise, 150 minutes of moderate aerobic exercise, or a combination of the two each week. The orders guide distributing out this exercise over the course of a week. At least 300 minutes per week are advised to promote even greater health benefits and help with weight loss or

maintaining weight loss. But even a little bit of exercise is beneficial. The cumulative effects of being active throughout the day can be beneficial to your health.

• Weight lifting. At least twice a week, perform strength-training exercises for all the major muscle groups.

The following are examples of the types of activities that are included in the program. Running, strenuous yard work and aerobic dancing are examples of activities that qualify as vigorous aerobic exercise. Use of weight machines, your own body weight, heavy bags, resistance tubing or paddles in the water, or exercises like rock climbing can all be considered forms of strength training.

You might need to increase your moderate aerobic activity even more if you want to lose weight, achieve certain fitness goals, or reap additional benefits.

Always consult your doctor before beginning a new exercise regimen, particularly if you have any concerns about your fitness, haven't worked out in a while, or suffer from chronic conditions like heart disease, diabetes, or arthritis.

You probably make a commitment to an exercise program at least once a year. But if the follow-through has been a challenge for you, you're definitely not alone. But there are so many good reasons to reaffirm your commitment and follow through.

Everybody loses momentum for a different reason. The bottom line is that you can start a fitness routine at any time if getting fit is something you value. In less time than it takes to scroll through your Facebook feed, you can complete a full day's worth of exercise.

In fact, you could do it while watching television. If you adhere to the advice of groups like the American Council on Exercise (ACE), all you need is a total of 150 minutes of workout per week to recover your heart health and lower your risk of developing a variety of other diseases. It is entirely up to you when and how you incorporate these minutes into your daily activities.

Start today, then use these suggestions to help you incorporate exercise into your daily routine.

## CREATE A SMART OBJECTIVE.

A smart goal is one that is time-bound, relevant, specific, measurable, and attainable (met by a deadline and done in a certain amount of time)

Setting goals aids in providing structure and focus for your desired outcomes. Achieving goals is rewarding, and momentum is boosted, according to fitness experts. Simply focus on the "attainable" portion of this equation. Setting an impossible goal only sets you up for failure. Instead of stimulating yourself to exercise daily for 30 minutes every day of the week when on some days you can't even get in 15, look at your schedule and find two days where you can really boost your workout time to 30 minutes. You will eventually reach your weekly goal of 150 minutes if everything adds up.

**Vow to increase your daily step count**
Public health professionals have urged Americans to walk 10,000 steps per day for almost ten years. People who walk 5 miles or more per day, which equals the

10,000-mile mark, are categorized as "active." "Highly active" people log 12,500 steps daily.

Even if losing weight isn't your primary objective, you should strive to increase your daily mileage in order to improve or maintain general health.

**Make being fit a way of life, not a trend.**

Many people make the error of working hard to achieve their fitness goals but then giving up afterward. They do not view fitness as a way of life, but rather as a means to an end. Weight gain and health issues may result from this. You won't experience the long-term advantages of consistent exercise if you don't consider fitness to be a lifestyle choice.

Yes, short-term weight loss or maintenance is possible with exercise. However, leading an active lifestyle has long-term advantages. It can lower your risk of developing potential health issues, such as high blood pressure, diabetes, heart disease, and obesity.

It's never too late to start exercising because it helps with health and well-being.

**Daily Exercise Is Allowed**

Your weekly routine should include exercise because it is so beneficial to your life. It's essential for maintaining fitness, enhancing general well-being, and reducing your risk of health issues, particularly as you get older.

In general, though, you don't have to work out every day, especially if you're working hard or pushing yourself to your limits.

You'll be fine if you choose to engage in some sort of moderate-intensity exercise each day. You must always pay attention to your body and refrain from pushing it past its limits.

Continue reading to learn how much exercise you should be getting, as well as some tips for working with a trainer.

How much is ideal?

When planning a workout schedule, a weekly day of rest is frequently advised, but occasionally you might feel the urge to exercise every day.

Working out every day is fine as long as you're not overdoing it or becoming obsessed with it.

Make sure you enjoy it without being too hard on yourself, especially when you're sick or injured.

Take a look at the aims you want to work out every day. Do a lighter or shorter version of your workout on the day that would normally be a rest day if you find that taking a day off makes it difficult to get back on track and maintain motivation.

A general guideline is to engage in 30 minutes per day of moderate exercise, adding up to at least 150 minutes per week. Alternately, aim for at least 75 minutes per week of vigorous exercise.

**Different Exercises**

Aim for at least 45 minutes of exercise each day to help you reach your fitness, health, or weight loss objectives. Include some sort of high-intensity exercise, like running or plyometric.

You can take a day off in between workouts if you're doing intense cardio or weightlifting, or you can alternate between working out different parts of your body on different days. Alter your routine instead of engaging in strenuous exercise every day.

**Longer vs. shorter**
It is preferable to perform a brief workout every day as opposed to one or two lengthy workouts per week. Similarly to this, it's better to engage in brief bursts of activity throughout the day rather than skip a workout entirely when you don't have time for one.

Exercises you should do on a regular basis Include each of the following four types of exercise in your routine to reap the most benefits, including a lower risk of injury:
• To increase overall fitness, do endurance exercises that increase your breathing and heart rate. Jogging, swimming, and dancing are some examples.
Strong training benefits you control your weight while developing muscle and firming up your bones. Exercises with confrontation bands, bodyweight training, and weightlifting are a few examples.
• Balance exercises facilitate daily motions while enhancing stability and preventing falls. Tai chi, balance drills, and standing yoga poses are a few examples.
• Flexibility exercises reduce physical pain and enhance posture, mobility, and range of motion. Stretches, yoga, and Pilates are some examples.

**Benefits**
Regular exercise has positive effects on all facets of your life as well as your general well-being. Observe the following advantages of exercise:
- Mood Enhancer

You might increase your energy, drive, and mood. You'll probably accomplish more in every area of your life, which will make you feel good about yourself.
Relaxation
Overall stress reduction can result in feelings of relaxation, restful sleep, and boosted confidence.

- Sociable Hour

The social aspect of group exercise allows you to meet up with friends or make new ones in a cheap and healthy way. Consider working out with a friend in the outdoors, which has its own advantages.

- Cognitive Process

Exercise improves mental clarity and cognitive function. It can help you cultivate mindfulness and make room for novel thoughts and ideas.

- Condition Control

Numerous health conditions, including cardiovascular disease, type 2 diabetes, high blood pressure, metabolic syndrome, certain types of cancer, arthritis, falls, depression, and anxiety, can be prevented or managed with regular exercise.
Regular exercise supports weight loss and helps prevent regaining lost weight if you're trying to lose weight.

**Remain inspired**
You can naturally apply the drive, discipline, and determination you gain from setting goals and following a plan to achieve them in other areas of your life.
Working out every day is fine if you're working toward weight loss goals or completing a challenge that involves a daily workout.

Consider different ways to stand up and start moving.
Keep track of or write down how much time you spend
sitting each day or each week. Make every effort to cut
this time down. Think about the following:
• Get off the train a few stops early and walk the
remaining distance.
• Work at a standing desk.
• Swap out passive, sedentary activities for active ones.
• If you must sit for prolonged periods, stand up at least
five minutes every hour. Try brisk walking, stationary
jogging, or standing exercises like jumping jacks, lunges,
or arm circles.

**Cautions**
There are a few safety precautions to take if you exercise
frequently or daily.
Daily exercise can result in burnout, fatigue, and
injuries. You might completely give up on your fitness
regimen as a result of any one of these factors.
Any new exercise routine should be started slowly, then
the duration and intensity should be gradually increased.
Recognize your body. If you encounter: Reduce the
intensity of your workouts.
• Pains and aches
• Excruciating muscle pain; feeling queasy; cramping;
nausea; and dizziness

## THE BEST METHODS FOR STAYING IN SHAPE AFTER 40

It's never too late to start living a healthier lifestyle and
reap the rewards of physical fitness.

According to the study's authors, increasing physical activity later in life has the same protective effect against cancer, cardiovascular disease, and all-cause mortality as doing so from adolescence through adulthood.
A total of 150 minutes per week of moderate activity, such as housework or gardening, or 75 minutes per week of vigorous activity, such as brisk walking, running, swimming, or aerobics, was found to reduce risks the best for both younger and older participants.
The benefits of staying active into old age go beyond those revealed by the study.
Improved strength and function as well as improved balance and fall prevention can be advantageous for older populations.
There are some important factors to take into consideration for people over 40 who are starting or returning to a fitness routine.

**Getting fit gradually**
To reduce risk as much as possible, the study's weekly activity recommendations must be met, but doing so gradually is necessary to prevent injury.
The top way for getting in shape
Specific exercises and a positive attitude are the two main components of getting in shape after 40.
After easing into fitness, people over 40 should aim to do the following regularly:
• 30 minutes per day of light to moderate aerobic exercise (100 steps per minute)
• balance exercises at least two days a week, three days a week, with all major muscle groups

Furthermore, focus on setting your mentality toward
success.
He has found that "building a motivational platform
anchored by the most valuable relationships in your life,
like your spouse, partner, children, grandchildren, or
career, is the best way to get in shape after 40."
When it comes to the effort and sacrifices involved in
leading a healthy lifestyle, "these relationships define
your personal 'why.'"

**Keep in mind that being healthy is a team sport.**
Maintaining an active social schedule that is focused on
healthy pursuits can keep you on track with your fitness
and health objectives.
Possible obstacles to success
What's stopping so many of us, when a new study says
it's never too late to improve our health outcomes?
Most people are only able to keep their New Year's
resolutions for a month or two, he claimed. I blame this
on a shaky cognitive link between their routine behavior
and their most important relationships.
In his own research with physically active men over 50,
he discovered that the key to success is the capacity to
make the link between one's dietary and exercise
regimens and their life goals.
"They understand that maintaining their health is
important if they are to achieve their goals.
Consequently, while getting fit after 40 involves easing
into specific exercises tailored to success, it's also about
understanding your underlying motivation for doing so.
It's the power of this positive association that keeps them
going when others give up.

# HOW TO GET MOTIVATED TO EXERCISE

We are all aware of the positive effects exercise and physical activity has on our bodies, minds, and spirits. But occasionally, the voice inside our heads that tells us to skip our workout or order takeout and work for a few more hours, wins.

When this occurs, it may be challenging to stick to your plan to prioritize fitness and visit the gym.

When that happens, having a list of inspirational advice can help you maintain consistency. We've put together a list of doable strategies to keep you inspired and on track to achieve your fitness objectives.

**General advice**

1. Establish your "why"

You can't always rely on outside factors to motivate you, like a vacation. Having a personal or emotional investment in your objectives comes from knowing your "why" for exercising.

2. Choose a cause.

Whether you're an avid Cross Fitter, runner, or walker, picking a cause to compete for can really inspire you. Numerous contests are held to raise money for causes such as Alzheimer's research, cancer research or funding for families, cystic fibrosis research, suicide prevention, and diabetes research and advocacy.

3. Always keep a backup plan.

Put a change of workout attire and a pair of shoes in a "just in case" bag and keep it in your car. When plans change, be prepared with an alternative workout, such as a walking route by your place of employment.

4. Adhere to the "3 x 10 rule"

Lacking time? No issue. Walk for 10 minutes three times per day. You can get a full-body workout by substituting a few squats, pushups, and crunches for your evening stroll. All of these brief exercises quickly add up and significantly reduce the amount of time you spend exercising each week.

5. Post-it strength

Sticky notes should be marked with encouraging phrases about exercising. Put them up on your computer at work, bathroom mirror, or alarm clock. They will act as an ongoing reminder to look after your health.

6. Utilize social media.

Instead of taking selfies and checking in every day, use social media to keep up with your fitness goals.

According to one study, participating in online groups can help you stick to an exercise routine because of the encouragement, accountability, and even friendly competition.

**Tips for working out alone**

7. Add the event to your calendar.

Choose the exercise you'll perform, the duration, and the location. Next, dedicate 10 minutes to schedule your weekly activities. Regular exercise is encouraged by incorporating physical activity into daily activities.

8. Simply unable to refuse your favorite TV show? Hop on the treadmill or other cardio equipment, turn on the TV, and watch the time fly by. Even better, develop the practice of only watching your preferred program when you are working out.

9. Pick a time.

You might be motivated to get out of bed and start moving in the morning by training for a race or other special event. Look for a training opportunity that is a few months away. Sign up and pay the entry fee to commit, then start working.

10. Participate in a challenge.

There is a challenge for everything. The list includes the plank challenge, the daily exercise challenge, and the squat challenge. What is good news? You won't have any trouble finding multiple challenges to join and complete because there are so many to choose from.

**Advice for Early Birds**

11. Wear your clothes to bed

Yes, this ruse actually works! Try wearing them to bed if hanging your clothes out at night isn't enough of a motivator.

12. Place your alarm away from people.

If you're a sleeper, you need to set your alarm clock on the other side of your room. You are compelled to leave your bed as a result. You are halfway through your workout if you are already dressed.

13. Assemble your team

Having a friend waiting for you makes working out much simpler. It's a good idea to bring a camera if you're going to the beach. Plus, finding a fitness buddy increases the amount of exercise you do.

14. Take podcasts to heart

Pick a podcast you've been meaning to check out, and only play it while you exercise. When going to the gym doesn't sound all that appealing, this gives you something to look forward to.

**Advice for At-Home Exercise**

15. Make a place.

You can improve your mindset and reduce distractions that could be a real motivation killer by designating a space in your home or apartment for exercise. You can create a sacred space in spare bedrooms, or basements, or even by dividing off a corner of the living room to do burpees or practice yoga.

16. Use a fitness app.

Numerous fitness apps offer exercises like yoga and Pilates as well as bodyweight circuits and high-intensity interval training. Choose one app and set up daily.

17. Workouts that concentrate on various fitness objectives. Cardio on Monday, yoga on Tuesday, strength training on Wednesday, and so forth are a few examples.

18. Move your phone to a different room.

When you're trying to work out, texts and emails from your boss are a motivation killer. Put your phone in a room far from where you're exercising to avoid losing motivation midway through a set of air squats.

**Advice for Regular Exercisers**

18. Lunchtime exercise

Log off, stand up, and move around! Request a walk from a coworker or visit the gym for a quick lunchtime workout. If exercise is a convenient part of your day, you're more likely to do it.

19. Go outside of the gym

Anywhere and at any time is a good place to exercise. Perform 25 squats each time you ascend the stairs. While

making calls or brushing your teeth while moving,
balance on one leg.
20. Be creative
One exercise program may be effective short-term but
not long-term. Change up your workouts from time to
time to keep your motor running strong. It's a good idea
to rotate through various fitness classes and forms of
resistance and cardio training each week.
21. Ensure adequate rest.
Your body may experience damage if you exercise daily.
Make sure one of the days of the week that you exercise
the most, if not every day, is set aside for active rest.
Overtraining can result from doing something too much
and leave you feeling defeated.

**Advice for the post-work group**
22. Before leaving for home, work out
Find a nearby track, gym, or hiking trail that you can
visit before leaving for the day. When you get to work,
change into your workout attire and head straight there.
No detours for grocery or dry cleaning stops.
23. Consider small steps
Sometimes it seems completely impossible to exercise
after a long day. Tell yourself that you'll just get dressed
and perform a 10-minute warm-up before you even
consider going home, rather than giving up before you've
even begun. There's a good chance that once you start
moving, you'll want to keep going.
24. Follow your passion
After work, working out should give you more energy
and help you forget about the day. You can stay

motivated more frequently by choosing activities and workouts that you enjoy and look forward to.

## ADVICE FOR WEIGHT LOSS

1. Set modest objectives.
Small goals consistently outperform larger ones when it comes to weight loss. Start by setting daily, weekly, and monthly goals before aiming to reach your objective.
2. Rim yourself with individuals who share your opinions.
It's difficult to lose weight, let's face it. But if you live with people who have bad eating and exercise habits, it will be very difficult to try to lose weight. To retain yourself on track, choose your friends wisely and relate with individuals who have related aims.
Make your eating plan effective for you, number.
 3. You may want to reconsider your current plan if you find yourself frequently changing the menu or packing food to stay on your diet.
In the long run, it is not advantageous to have an "all or nothing" mentality. A lifestyle change that gives you the freedom to live without planning your day around a diet is necessary to lose weight and keep it off.
4. Always bring a take-out container home.
Ask the server to bring a to-go container with your meal when you're out to eat. Put the other half of the meal in the container right away, and then just consume what is on your plate. You not only reduce your calorie intake but also have lunch prepared for the following day.

1. A weekly day of meal preparation
Every week, set aside a day to go shopping, and prepare, and cook at least two or three lunches. Several items for meals on the go include:
• Chicken breast
• Salad
• Fruit
• Veggies (Brown rice)
• Sweet potatoes;
 • Burrito bowl ingredients
To make it easier for you to grab and go when leaving the house, divide each meal into smaller containers.
2. Concentrate on adding, not subtracting
Instead of eliminating everything you believe to be unhealthy, concentrate on including foods like fruits and vegetables that may be missing from your diet.
3. All week, attempt one new process.
Choose one new healthy recipe to prepare that includes a lean protein source such as chicken or fish, vegetables, a complex carbohydrate, healthy fats, and fruit for dessert.
4. Replace sugary beverages with flavored water.
Instead of drinking soda, juice, or fizzy water that has added sugar, try flavoring plain water with some natural flavors. Consider mixing one of these into your water for a tasty and refreshing beverage:
• Cucumbers
• Strawberries
• Oranges
• Lime
• Mint

# CHAPTER 6

## LIVING A HEALTHY LIFESTYLE

Most people define "healthy living" as having both physical and mental health that is balanced and works well together. Physical and mental health are frequently intertwined, making changes in either one (for the better or worse) immediately impact the other. As a result, some of the advice will include recommendations for "healthy living" on the emotional and mental levels.

Although it is not intended to be exhaustive, this chapter will include the key elements that are thought to be a part of a lifestyle that promotes good health. Its purpose is to provide readers with advice on how they can enhance or improve actions in their lives to have a healthy lifestyle. The chapter will also include some advice on avoiding behaviors (the don'ts) that promote unhealthy living in addition to suggestions for what people should do to lead healthy lives.

**Eating Well (Diet and Nutrition)**

All individuals must eat food in order to grow and sustain a healthy body, but as infants, children (kids), teenagers, young adults, adults, and seniors, we have different nutritional needs. For instance, until they gradually mature and start consuming more solid foods, infants may need to be fed every four hours. They eventually adapt to eating three times a day as young children, which is more typical. The majority of parents are aware that children, teenagers, and young adults frequently snack in between meals. Snacking is often done by adults and elders as well, so it is not just a practice among this age set.

## ADVICE FOR REGULAR HEALTHY EATING

• Consume three balanced meals per day—breakfast, lunch, and dinner—and keep in mind that dinner does not necessarily need to be the largest meal of the day.
• Healthy foods like fruits, vegetables, whole grains, and fat-free or low-fat milk products should make up the majority of your diet.
• Include lean meats, poultry, fish, beans, eggs, and nuts in your diet, with a focus on the latter two.
• Opt for foods that are low in saturated fats, trans fats, cholesterol, salt (sodium), and added sugars; pay attention to the ingredients list because the first items on the list have the highest concentrations of ingredients.
• Watch your portion sizes; only consume as much as is necessary to satiate hunger.
• Healthy snacks, which should include things like fruit, whole grains, or nuts to satisfy hunger and prevent excessive weight gain, are acceptable in moderation.
• Due to their high-calorie content, avoid sodas and drinks with added sugar. Diet beverages may also not be a wise choice as they can increase a person's appetite and food intake in some cases.
• To prevent weight gain and gastro esophageal reflux disease, avoid eating a substantial meal just before bed.
• Eating while upset or depressed won't make them feel better and might even make their problems worse.

• Steer clear of rewarding kids with sugary treats; doing so could develop into a habit that lasts a lifetime.
• In the summer, especially on hot days, stay away from heavy meals.
• Vegetarians should check with their doctors to make sure they are getting enough vitamins, minerals, and iron in their diet. A vegetarian lifestyle has been promoted for a healthy lifestyle and weight loss.
• The majority of harmful bacteria and other pathogens are destroyed when food is cooked (above 165 F). If you choose to eat uncooked foods, such as fruits or vegetables, you should thoroughly wash them with running-treated (safe to drink) tap water right before eating.
• Steer clear of any type of meat that is raw or undercooked.

**Advice for unique circumstances:**
• Those who have diabetes should follow the aforementioned advice, monitor their blood glucose levels as instructed, and make every effort to maintain daily blood glucose levels as close to normal as they can.
• People who work atypical hours (night shifts, college students, and military personnel) should try to stick to a breakfast, lunch, and dinner schedule with little snacking.
• Those who prepare food should refrain from frying anything in grease.
• Seek medical advice as soon as possible if you are unable to control your weight, and food intake, or if you have diabetes and are unable to control your blood glucose levels.

• People trying to lose weight (body fat) should avoid all fatty and sugary foods and eat mostly vegetables, fruits, and nuts.

## PHYSICAL AND MENTAL HEALTH BENEFITS OF EXERCISE

**Physical wellbeing**

People are made to use their bodies and inactivity results in unhealthy living. Exercise are main contributors to a healthy lifestyle. Obesity, weakness, lack of endurance, and general ill health are all symptoms of unhealthy living and may promote the onset of disease.

Regular exercise can improve balance, flexibility, and endurance, prevent and reverse age-related declines in muscle mass and strength, and reduce the risk of falls in the elderly. Coronary heart disease, stroke, diabetes, obesity, and high blood pressure can all be avoided with regular exercise. • Regular fitness can help people with chronic arthritis improve their ability to perform daily activities like driving, climbing stairs, and opening jars. Regular fitness can also help people with osteoporosis by strengthening bones.

• Regular exercise can help control body weight and in some people lead to fat loss.

• Regular exercise can help improve mood, reduce stress and anxiety, increase self-esteem and self-confidence, and improve overall mental health.

**Guidelines for consistent exercise:**

• While it's advised to exercise for 30 minutes each day, most days of the week are when you'll see the biggest health benefits (brisk walking counts).
• You can divide your workout into smaller, 10-minute sessions.
• Begin slowly and increase your activity level gradually to prevent injury, excessive soreness, or fatigue. Build up to daily moderate to the vigorous exercise of 30 to 60 minutes over time.
• Anyone can start exercising at any age. Even frail, elderly people (between 70 and 90 years old) can strengthen their bodies and balance with exercise.
• Almost all forms of exercise are beneficial for everyone, including resistance training, water aerobics, walking, swimming, weight lifting, and yoga.
• Children need to be active, and playing outside is a good place to start.
• Children's sports can be great ways to get exercise, but it's important to avoid overdoing some of them (for example, throwing too many pitches in baseball may harm a joint like an elbow or shoulder).
• Strenuous exercise may leave a person exhausted and sore, but if pain develops, stop exercising until the cause of the pain is identified; the person may need to seek medical assistance and advice about whether to continue the exercise.

Most people don't need a medical checkup to start doing moderate exercise like walking. However, the following people should speak with a doctor before starting a more intense exercise program:
• People who are over 40 or over 50; those who have heart or lung disease; those who have arthritis,

osteoporosis, or asthma; those who get tired easily or experience shortness of breath when exerting themselves;
• People who smoke, have high blood cholesterol, high blood pressure, or have a family history of coronary heart disease or early-onset heart attacks, among other conditions that increase the risk of developing coronary heart disease.
• People who are severely obese

**Physical inactivity and a lack of exercise have the following negative effects:**
• Lack of exercise and physical inactivity is linked to type II diabetes mellitus (also known as maturity or adult-onset, non-insulin-dependent diabetes).
• Heart disease and certain malignancies are linked to physical inactivity and a lack of exercise.
• Lack of exercise and physical inactivity can lead to weight growth.

## MENTAL HEALTH

Healthy living encompasses emotional or mental health in addition to physical health. The methods individuals may assist their mental health and well-being are as follows.

**Procedures for improving mental health:**
• Get enough sleep every night. The CDC recommends the following amounts for each age group (naps included): 12–18 hours for infants and toddlers, 14–15 hours for children aged 3–11 months, 12–18 hours for children aged 1–3 years, 11–13 hours for children aged

3–5 years, 10–11 hours for children aged 5–10 years, 8.5–9.5 hours for children aged 10–17 years, and 7-9 hours for people aged 18 and over. Older folks need around 7-9 hours of sleep, but they do not sleep as deeply and may wake up early in the morning or at night. Hence, naps (as kids require) enable them to accrue the 7-9 hours of sleep necessary.

• At least a few times a week, go for a stroll and think about what you see and hear.

• Attempt novel things often (eat new food, try a different route to work, go to a new museum display).

• Do mental exercises (read, do a puzzle occasionally during the week).

• Try to give a task your whole attention for one to many hours at a time, then take a break and do something enjoyable (walk, exercise, short nap).

• Schedule some time to chat with others about various topics.

• Make an effort to set aside time each week for leisure activities (hobby, sport).

• Practice saying "no" when anything comes up that you don't want to do or participate in.

• Have fun.

• Let yourself take pride in all of your accomplishments, no matter how minor (develop contentment).

• Develop a social support system; those who have it tend to have better lives.

• If you feel sad, have suicidal thoughts, or are thinking about hurting yourself or others, get assistance and guidance as soon as possible.

• Even if a person feels "better," they should not stop taking medication for mental health disorders until they have spoken with the doctor who prescribed it about their condition (s).

Another important aspect of well-being is avoidance behavior. Some of the key things to avoid are listed below for those looking to lead a healthy lifestyle. Avoid using tobacco.

According to the National Cancer Institute, tobacco smoking is the most avoidable disease and cause of death in the United States (NCI). In the United States, it was projected that 443,000 fatalities in 2010 were related to tobacco usage.

• Put an end to tobacco use (it takes about 15 years of nonsmoking behavior to achieve a "normal" risk level for heart disease for those that smoke).

• Quit chewing tobacco if you want to prevent oral cancer.

**Consequences of tobacco usage include:**

• Smoking causes or aggravates a significant number of malignancies in the United States. Smoking causes 80% of lung cancer deaths in women and 90% of lung cancer deaths in men. Lung, mouth, lip, tongue, esophagus, kidney, and bladder cancers are brought on by smoking. Moreover, it raises the risk of lung cancer in those exposed to asbestos and the risk of bladder cancer in people exposed to certain organic compounds used in the textile, leather, rubber, dye, and other organic chemical industries.

• Smoking results in atherosclerotic artery disease, which causes the arteries to stiffen and narrow. This condition may cause heart attacks, strokes, and reduced blood flow to the lower limbs. According to estimates, tobacco smoking causes 20% to 30% of coronary heart disease in the US. Also, it raises the risk of heart attacks in those who are obese, have high cholesterol, has uncontrolled hypertension, and have sedentary lifestyles.

• Cigarette smoking causes pneumonia in people with chronic lung disease, which is thought to account for 20% of chronic lung illnesses in the United States, including emphysema and chronic bronchitis. In 2011, the CDC projected that smoking was to blame for 90% of fatalities from chronic obstructive pulmonary disease (COPD).

Smoking during pregnancy increases the risk of low birth weight, and secondhand smoke may exacerbate asthma in children and cause middle ear infections (otitis media), coughing, wheezing, bronchitis, and pneumonia in infants. Lung cancer may also be brought on by passive smoking, sometimes known as secondhand smoke.

**Advice for giving up tobacco:**

• Smoking cessation is challenging because the nicotine in tobacco is addicting. Some smokers are able to stop "cold turkey," but the majority must make a serious, lifelong commitment and make an average of six tries before they are successful.

• Methods for quitting smoking include behavior modification, counseling, the use of nicotine skin patches (Transderm Nicotine), nicotine chewing gum (Nicorette Gum), and oral drugs like bupropion (Zyban). Limit your alcohol intake.

**Unfavorable effects of heavy alcohol use:**

In the United States, liver cirrhosis is mostly brought on by long-term, excessive alcohol usage.

• Liver cirrhosis may result in liver cancer and cause internal hemorrhaging, fluid buildup in the abdomen, easy bleeding and bruising, muscular wasting, mental disorientation, infections, and in severe instances, coma, and renal failure.

• In the United States, 40% to 50% of fatal car accidents include alcohol.

• Drowning, burns, and house accidents are among the leading causes of injury and death that result from alcohol consumption.

**Advice for reducing alcohol consumption:**

Alcoholism may be treated in a variety of ways. Yet acknowledging there is a problem and pledging to deal with the alcoholism issue is an essential first step in the recovery process. One successful therapy is the 12-step approach to self-help that Alcoholics Anonymous developed. Psychologists and other associated experts have created programs to assist people in better managing their emotions and avoiding actions that might result in binge drinking. Family members' understanding and support are often essential for long-term healing. After an acute or chronic intoxication, medication may help with withdrawal symptoms and the avoidance of relapses.

## STEER CLEAR OF RISKY SEXUAL CONDUCT.

The development of sexually transmitted diseases including gonorrhea, syphilis, herpes, or HIV infection may result from high-risk sexual conduct. High-risk sexual conduct is also known to transmit human papillomavirus infection, which may lead to cervical cancer in women and other anogenital malignancies in

both men and women. The following are some examples of high-risk sexual behaviors:
• Multiple sex partners
• Sexual partners who have a history of:
• Use of intravenous drugs
• Venereal illness (sexually transmitted diseases or STDs)
**Negative effects of high-risk sexual conduct include:**
• The spread of sexually transmitted illnesses such as HIV (chlamydia, gonorrhea, syphilis, genital herpes)
• Hepatitis B transmission (sex accounts for 50% of hepatitis B infections) and, in rare cases, hepatitis C transmission
• The spread of the human papillomavirus (HPV), which may lead to an genital cancers (most often uterine cervix cancer) and genital warts,
• An unintended pregnancy
• Avoid unprotected sex (sex without barriers like a condom) outside of a committed, monogamous relationship, according to these prevention tips.
Use a condom if you intend to have sex but are uncertain of your partner's health.

## STAY AWAY FROM OTHER RISKY ACTIVITIES.

• Avoid high-risk activities like
• Driving when intoxicated or high
• Driving when exhausted; • Careless driving, speeding, and "road rage;"
• Cell phone use, texting, or other chores while driving

• Failure to wear a helmet while riding a motorcycle or bicycle;
• Unsafe storage and handling of firearms and other weapons in one's possession.
• Smoking in bed Negative effects of risky behaviors: Motorbike accidents are a significant source of severe head injuries.
• Guns and weapons account for a considerable share of teenage fatalities related to male suicide and murder.
• Smoking in bed may result in burn injuries and death.
• Use seat restraints on all passengers when driving, in both the front and back seats.
• Never drive after drinking.
• If you're sleep deprived, don't drive.
• While driving, put down unneeded distractions and pay attention to the road and other traffic (avoid texting, talking on cell phones, eating, applying makeup, or other distractions).
• Whether riding a motorbike or bicycle, always wear a helmet. Wearing a helmet decreases major head injuries by 75% and motorcycle accident mortality by 30%.
• Get the right instruction in the handling and storage of weapons and ammunition.
• Use smoke alarms; avoid smoking in bed.
• Use sunscreen, brimmed hats, protective clothes, and other sun protection measures to prevent sunburns and exposure to the sun.
The U.S. FDA (Food and Drug Administration) announced new guidelines for sunscreens to follow beginning in 2012. Sunscreens have undergone adjustments. The FDA now advises that an effective sunscreen has an SPF of 30 or higher and offers UVA

and UVB protection (protection against ultraviolet waves of types A and B). Most of the time, sunscreen has to be reapplied every two hours, always after swimming.

Diet for a Heart-Healthy Heart: 25 Items You Should Consume

Your heart is an exactly improved appliance. You must offer it with heart-healthy fuel to keep it operating at peak effectively. So, you have to make a nutritious diet your priority. Certain meals are excellent for your heart, but how do you choose?

The risk of cardiovascular illness, such as coronary artery disease, which may cause a heart attack or stroke, can be reduced by choosing the proper nutritious meals.

## FOODS FOR STABILIZING YOUR BLOOD VESSELS AND HEART

These are the top 25 foods for preserving your blood vessels and heart. Discover the top nutrients that maintain a healthy heartbeat and get menu ideas for including these foods in your everyday meals.

- Salmon

Salmon contains significant amounts of omega-3 fatty acids, which may reduce your risk of arrhythmias, lower triglyceride levels, inhibit the development of arterial plaque, and modestly lower blood pressure. All week, two meals of omega-3-rich foods like salmon are recommended by the American Heart Association. A cooked fish serving is 3.5 ounces.

Salmon is a food with numerous uses. Add it to your salads for a protein boost or grill it with a rub or marinade. You can also chop it and use it in a pasta dish with fat-free marinara sauce.

Salmon: Wild vs. Farmed

Does the method use to grow your salmon affect how much omega-3 it contains? Both farm-raised and wild-caught salmon is now available at many supermarket shops. It turns out that salmon produced on farms tends to have greater overall fat as well as omega-3 fat. Although farmed salmon includes more saturated fat than flank steak does, the quantity is still about half as high.

- Flaxseed (ground)

Together with soluble and insoluble fiber, ground flaxseed also contains omega-3 fatty acids. It keeps one of the uppermost absorptions of lignans, which are antioxidants and plant estrogens.

You can add ground flaxseed to almost everything you typically eat and it's simple to integrate into your diet. You may add it to muffin batter, low-fat yogurt, morning cereal, smoothies, and muffin tops.

What is Flaxseed oil?

Omega-3s abound in flaxseed oil, however, they are of the less potent ALA kind (alpha-linoleic acid). To convert ALA into omega-3, specific enzymes are required, and your body only has a little quantity of these enzymes. This implies that at most 15% of the omega-3s in flaxseed oil will be transformed into their most beneficial forms. So although you surely do receive some benefits, it may be less than your supplement label indicates.

- Oatmeal

Oatmeal is a wonderful morning item and another rich source of those omega-3 fatty acids. With 4 grams in all cup, it is also a fiber capital. Other diets included in it include magnesium, potassium, and iron.

With some fresh berries on top, oatmeal becomes an even more heart-healthy breakfast option. Try making whole rolled oats into a turkey burger meatloaf, fat-free oatmeal cookies, or oat bread.

- Kidney or Black Beans

The familiar playground refrains, "Beans, beans, excellent for your heart," is used. That seems to be true! Beans are a excessive basis of doable fiber, omega-3 fatty acids, B-complex vitamins, niacin, folate, magnesium, and calcium.

Beans have a lot of uses. You may incorporate them in soups, stews, or salads. Or use them to prepare dinner. Try black beans with avocado on a whole-grain pita tostada, or fill bell peppers with them after mixing them with corn and onions. Cucumber, fresh corn, onions, and peppers are join in a salad with canned kidney beans; it is then dressed with olive oil and apple cider vinegar. Instead, joint black beans and kidney beans to produce a flavorful, wholesome vegetarian chili.

- Almonds

Nuts have been demonstrated to reduce blood cholesterol. Almonds are a fantastic option for a nut that is good for your heart. These include heart-healthy monounsaturated and polyunsaturated fats, vitamin E, magnesium, calcium, fiber, and plant omega-3 fatty acids.

Almonds are quite simple to consume; you may sprinkle them over yogurt, salads, or as a trail mix snack. You may use them in cooking as well. Almonds without salt provide further heart protection.

Just make sure that your almonds are raw or dry roasted (as opposed to oil roasted) and pay attention to portion quantities. Although heart-healthy, they contain a lot of fat, including some saturated fat. Almonds have many calories, more like other nuts, so a small bit goes a long way. It's preferable to consume them in moderation.

- Walnuts

Almonds and other tree nuts provide similar health benefits as walnuts. They include phytosterols, heart-healthy monosaturated and polyunsaturated fats, vitamin E, magnesium, folate, fiber, and plant omega-3 fatty acids.

Walnuts offer salads a robust crunch much as almonds provide. They go healthy with muffins and pancakes for breakfast.

While being heart-healthy, they contain a lot of fat and calories and should only be consumed in moderation. Be mindful of walnut portion proportions as you would with any nut. The palm of your hand should comfortably accommodate one serving of walnuts, which has roughly 200 calories.

- A red wine

Catechins are a set of flavonoids located in red wine, joint with the antioxidant resveratrol. Flavonoids may support avoid blood clots and support the health of your blood vessels. In the lab, resveratrol has been shown to have heart-healthy properties.

Have some wine with dinner or create a wine spritzer by combining wine and sparkling water to reduce calories while retaining many of the advantages.

But remember that the American Heart Association does not advise individuals to start drinking in order to just stave against heart disease. Alcohol use increases the likelihood of developing alcoholism and increases the risk of obesity, high blood pressure, stroke, breast cancer, suicide, and automobile accidents. Drink red wine sparingly (for example, one wine glass full with a meal).

- Tuna

The omega-3 fatty acids located in tuna. The level of omega-3s in tuna is fairly pleasant, while not being as great as that in salmon. Niacin, a vitamin that may increase the chances of survival for those who have had a heart attack, is also included in one serving of tuna and makes up nearly half of your daily needs.

A quick and filling lunchtime snack is tuna salad with little mayo. Tuna may be meshed for a nice meal as well as a fantastic salad accumulation.

Selecting tuna cans

One of the most regular consumed types of seafood in America is tuna in cans. Yet with so many options, selecting the best can also be challenging. The two most prevalent forms are white tuna, manufactured from albacore, and light tuna, created from lesser fish types (usually skipjack). White contains greater amounts of mercury, which is especially problematic for expectant mothers, but it also has more omega-3s.

Some tuna is traded in water, while others are sold in oil. Omega 3 fat is substantially more plenty in tuna in water. This is due to the fact that a significant amount of the omega 3 fat is lost when you drain the oil from the bowl.


- Tofu

A fantastic source of protein is tofu. Vegetarian food. Moreover, it is rich in minerals that are good for the heart, including niacin, folate, calcium, magnesium, and potassium.

Tofu is frequently called "bean curd" since it is formed from pressed soybean curd. It is simple to make and goes fine with essentially any meal.

Firm tofu should be thinly sliced and marinated for a few hours before grilling or adding to your favorite vegetable stir-fry. Use tofu instead of meat in pasta meals and add slices or cubes to salads for extra protein. You can also make a tofu, lettuce, and tomato sandwich on whole-grain bread.

Steer clear of processed tofu products.

While tofu has been demonstrated in several studies to have heart-protective characteristics, it relies on how you cook it. Even though it might be nutritious, tofu is not always surrounded by friends. It may be found in a lot of ultra-processed foods, which have been linked to cardiovascular disease and obesity. In 2017, the FDA revoked some of the heart health benefits of tofu products due to their usage in high-calorie processed meals.

- Dark Rice

Brown rice is a heart-healthy food choice in addition to being delicious. B-complex vitamins, magnesium, and fiber are all existing in Dark rice.

You can't go in mistake by including dark rice in almost any food. Microwaveable Dark rice with a few chopped vegetables bids a simple and fast meal. Make a stir-fry, add it to soups, combine it with some black beans or tofu, or try it icy in an avocado salad.

- nut milk

Is flavones, a kind of flavonoid, is present in soy milk, which is a rich source of nutrients. In comparison to animal milk, soy milk contains more protein, which may help reduce blood cholesterol levels and have other positive effects on the cardiovascular system.

Use soy milk in lieu of dairy milk in any dish, whether it be in a smoothie or your whole grain cereal.

- Blueberries

Berries are healthy for your body as a whole and your heart in particular. The antioxidants beta-carotene and lutein, the flavonoid anthocyanin, the polyphenol ellagic acid, the vitamins C and folate, calcium, magnesium, potassium, and fiber are all existing in large sizes in blueberries.

Berries are simple to have as a nourishing snack on their own, on top of cereal or pancakes, in a smoothie, as a sauce for low-fat yogurt, or as part of a salad.

- Carrots

Most people probably know carrots best for their carotenoid content. Carrots are an excellent source of alpha and gamma carotenes in addition to the well-known vitamin beta-carotene (carotenoids). Higher beta carotene levels have been linked in studies to a decreased risk of heart disease and stroke.

- Spinach

With beta-carotene, vitamins C and E, potassium, folate, calcium, and fiber, spinach is a powerhouse of heart-healthy nutrients.
In place of lettuce, spinach works well as a salad dressing and as a filling for sandwiches. Also, you may smuggle some into fruit smoothies, add them to pizza, or include it into egg white omelets. Alternatively, for an added health benefit, add it to your pasta recipe.
Fresh or frozen spinach?
How long it's been sitting determines the answer. Freshly grown spinach includes more folate than frozen spinach, and according to some studies, folate may reduce your chance of developing heart disease. But there's a catch: the folate in fresh spinach deteriorates with time. Hence, frozen spinach could be healthier if your fresh spinach has been stored for a week in the fridge or has traveled great distances to get to your table.
Broccoli

Beta-carotene, vitamins C and E, potassium, folate, calcium, and fiber make broccoli a potent food.
Broccoli is delicious when added to soups, salads, vegetable dips, and dishes with brown rice. Increasing

your intake of broccoli is a certain strategy to boost the health of your heart.

- Sugar Potato

A great source of vitamins is sweet potatoes. In addition to containing vitamins A and C, sweet potatoes are also a unique low-fat source of vitamin E. Moreover, they include fiber, potassium, folate, calcium, and calcium, and when you eat their skins, you get even more fiber.
A sweet potato will taste good practically any way you cook it. Bake it entirely and add vegetables on top. For healthy fries, slice it into wedges and bake till crisp. For a soup that tastes velvety, purée sweet potatoes in a food processor. They are also delicious mashed up as a side dish.
Yams are nutritious, but sweet potatoes have more vitamins, minerals, and fiber.

- Red Bell peppers

For further information, please contact us.
Peppers taste great in salads and sandwiches, or you can slice them and eat them raw as a snack. To add flavor to sauces or main courses, roast or grill them for a substantial side dish.
Color matters when it comes to the heart-healthy compounds in bell peppers. For example, red peppers contain large amounts of beta-carotene. Yellow bells contain hardly little beta-carotene at all while being healthful in many other ways.

- Asparagus

Asparagus is a nutritious vegetable that includes beta-carotene, lutein, folate, fiber, and vitamins B and C.
A great heart-healthy side dish is asparagus. Sprinkle some balsamic vinaigrette on top and gently grill or steam the dish. Add to salads, stews, or casseroles to boost their nutritional value.

- Oranges

Oranges make the ideal snack. The antioxidant beta-cryptoxanthin, carotenoids like beta- and alpha-carotene and lutein, flavones (flavonoids), vitamin C, potassium, folate, and fiber are all present in them. They are also juicy and packed with these nutrients.
The fruit should be eaten whole since it tastes best that way. Orange slices may also be used in salads, yogurt, and even poultry recipes. Orange juice may also give some of the same advantages, but pound for pound you are better off eating the fruit whole.

- Tomatoes

With beta- and alpha-carotene, lycopene, lutein (carotenoids), vitamin C, potassium, folate, and fiber, tomatoes are a diverse, heart-healthy meal. Studies on lycopene in particular as a potential defense against cardiovascular disease are still lacking in clarity.
Tomatoes may be added raw to salads or sandwiches. They are the ideal complement to pasta recipes when cooked and produce fantastic sauces.

- Squash Acorn

Another heart-healthy meal is acorn squash, which also contains beta-carotene and lutein (carotenoids), the vitamins B complex and C, folate, calcium, magnesium, potassium, and fiber.

Acorn squash baked is a wonderful winter dish. Cut the squash in half, remove the seeds, and then fill it with brown rice and vegetables before roasting.

- Cantaloupe

Alpha-, beta-, and lutein (carotenoids), B-complex and C vitamins, folate, potassium, and fiber are all present in cantaloupe, a summertime staple that also has these heart-healthy elements.

Just cut a piece of cantaloupe and eat it whenever you like! Try blending some into a smoothie or combining them with other fruits to make a fresh fruit salad.

- Papaya

The carotenoids beta-carotene, beta-cryptoxanthin, and lutein are found in papaya. Together with folate, calcium, and potassium, it also includes the vitamins A and C in your diet.

Salmon, a heart-healthy food, pairs well with papaya. Try using it in a fruit salad, smoothie, Popsicle, salsa, or even on the grill.

- Dark Chocolate

Happy news Resveratrol, a heart-healthy antioxidant found in chocolate, as well as cocoa phenols, helps decrease blood pressure.

To gain the advantages, stick to dark chocolate with a 70% cocoa content or greater, and keep in mind that

moderation is crucial since chocolate is heavy in calories, fat, and sugar. You just need one serving.
Tea
Similar to red wine, tea contains catechins and flavonols that may prevent blood clots from developing and help preserve the health of your blood vessels. Particularly green tea has been praised for its anti-inflammatory qualities.
According to lengthy research involving more than 6,000 individuals, drinking tea may lower your chance of developing heart issues. Those who consumed 1-3 cups of tea each day had higher coronary calcium scores, according to the research. Coronary calcium may be a sign of future cardiac issues like a heart attack or stroke. Hot or cold tea is welcome. Add some lemon, maybe. Use hotter water and let the tea soak for at least three to five minutes if you want to extract additional antioxidants from it. Steer clear of sugar and cream since they contribute extra calories and fat.

# *FINAL SUMMARY*

An innovative method for achieving ideal weight reduction and health is the Galveston Diet. It blends Mediterranean diet principles with the most recent findings in a scientific study on nutrition, metabolism, and exercise. The end result is a complete regimen that may assist you in maintaining a healthy weight while also assisting you in losing weight. The diet has an emphasis on natural, unprocessed foods, restricts sugar and refined carbs, and promotes routine exercise. Also, it offers pointers on how to modify your way of life to support your health objectives. The Galveston Diet is a method of health and weight management that is sustainable and personalized for each person. It may assist you in achieving your health and weight reduction objectives with the proper dietary, activity, and lifestyle modifications.

The Galveston Diet emphasizes intermittent fasting since it is thought to promote weight reduction, control insulin levels, and enhance general health.

The Galveston Diet provides a complete strategy for long-term weight reduction and optimum health overall. It creates a regimen that may assist anybody in achieving their health and weight reduction objectives by fusing the most recent scientific research with Mediterranean principles. You may learn the key to long-term success with your health and weight loss by adhering to the program and making the essential lifestyle adjustments. Overall, the Galveston Diet offers a safe and effective strategy for women to lose weight and achieve optimum health. The Galveston Diet aims to help women in attaining and sustaining a healthy weight and improving their general health and well-being by embracing the concepts of the Mediterranean diet, intermittent fasting, and a low-carb, high-fat strategy.

www.ingramcontent.com/pod-product-compliance
Lightning Source LLC
Chambersburg PA
CBHW070739250726
48662CB00004B/1586